You *don't need* a Baker

DO IT YOURSELF WITH THESE DELICIOUS, EASY TO FOLLOW, RECIPES

SUZIANA BACHTIAR (BELLA)

Photography and recipes: Suziana Bachtiar
Editing and chief taster: Peter Wescombe
Layout and Design: Maria Azka

ISBN: 978-1-7635693-3-1
First published in Australia 2024
Copyright 2024 by Wescombe Publishing
All rights reserved

Contact information
  Facebook: bella chocolate cakes
  Email: suzianabella@gmail.com

Dedicated to Andra, Alvin, Aloka and my beautiful grandchildren. And to all the dear friends and lovers of my cakes in Bowen, Queensland

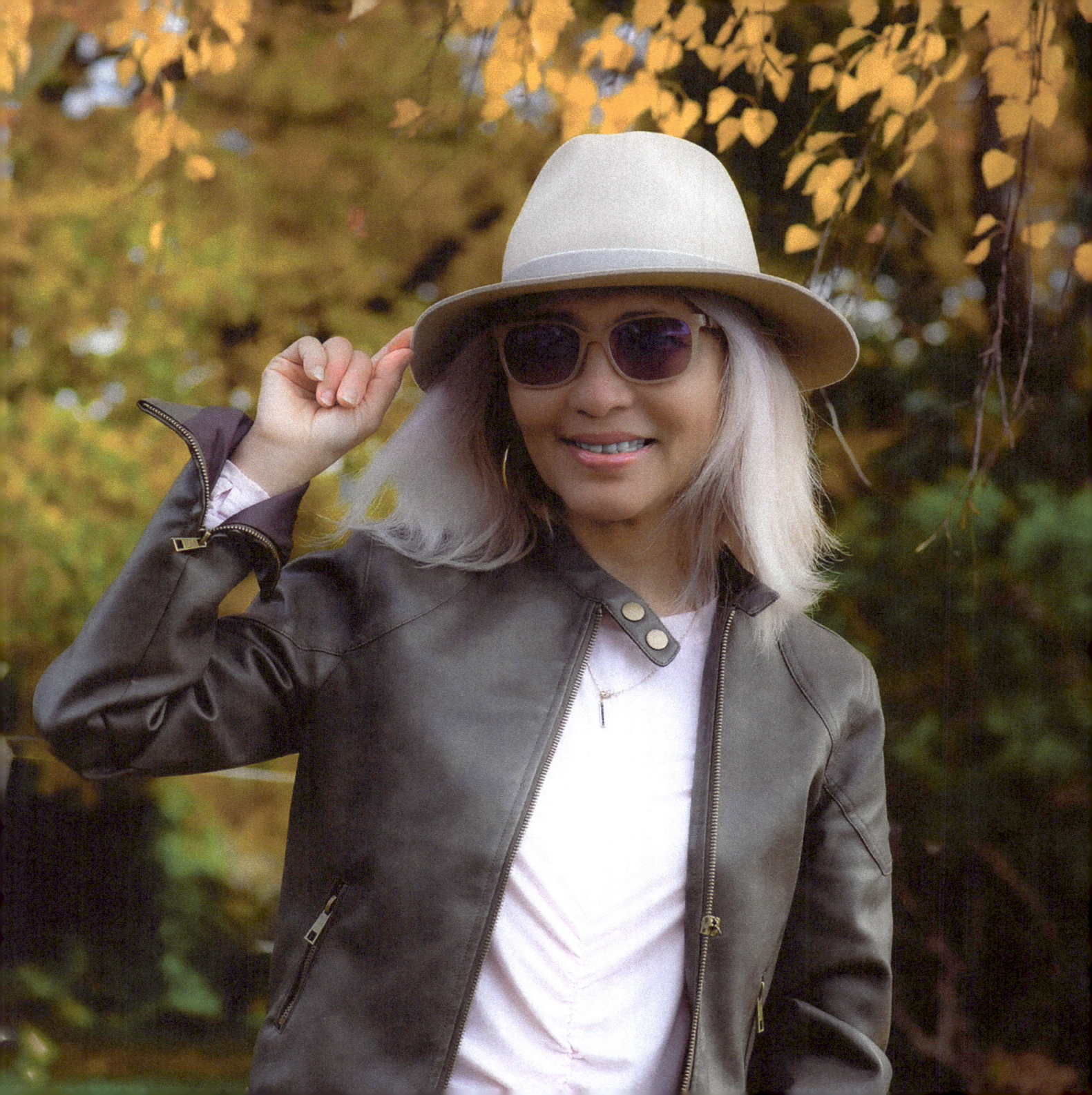

INTRODUCTION

I have always loved baking and cooking and spending time in the kitchen. It is more than just a hobby – it is a part of who I am. This passion, along with my curious nature and eagerness to learn, has motivated me to always be trying out new recipes and coming up with creative baking ideas. I have also been fortunate to have learned some recipes and baking skills from excellent bakers. I am passionate about both the science of baking as well as the freedom it offers to experiment

I first started out on my own food and cooking journey in in Ubud, Bali in 2015 when I opened my own **Holy Basil café**, catering to the vegan and vegetarian community. Later, after moving to Bowen, Qld, I found myself again drawn to the kitchen and baking. I received my first cake order after making my signature Black Forest cake. My partner at the time, took some of it to work to share with his mates who all loved it. One of them pulled out $40 and said "Can you get me $40 worth of that cake" I realized no one was making cakes like the way I make my Black Forest cake and other similar special cakes.

Shortly afterwards I started working at a local BP service station and there I had the good fortune of being able to promote and sell some of my cakes to the service station customers. From there the demand for my cakes increased quickly and I soon started my own full time business **Bella Chocolate Cakes**, catering to the people of Bowen and surrounding areas.

I later had the opportunity to run a small café for a large Aged Care centre in Bowen, specializing in baking customized birthday cakes, as well as other speciality foods and dishes for the elderly residents. What a wonderful privilege it was to be able to bring some good cheer and a smile to these precious elderly people for their birthdays and other special occasions

Since moving to Tasmania last year, I have been concerned for the many people who loved my cakes and baking and are no longer able to enjoy them, and the idea of creating **You Don't Need a Baker** was born. My vision for this book was to create a way for my many wonderful customers, as well as anyone else, to be able to make these cakes by themselves using simple, healthy ingredients, straight from their pantry, and without feeling they need a baker, or need to be an expert in the kitchen.

Feel free to try some of these wonderful recipes, and it is my hope that you will love and enjoy and have lots of fun in the process, as I do when I'm baking. It is my pleasure to offer this book to you

Cheers

Bella

Contents

CAKES

MOIST VANILLA GOODNESS	11
RICH BLACKFOREST CAKE	13
RED VELVET PERFECTION	17
LEMON AND POPPY SEED TREATS	21
RASPBERRY CAKE WITH WHITE CHOCOLATE GANACHE	23
CHOCOLATE GANACHE CAKE	25
PISTACHIO CAKE WITH A LEMON KISS	27
BUTTER CAKE	29
BANANA CHOCOLATE CAKE	31
CHOCOLATE ESPRESSO CAKE	33
BRAZILIAN SWEET CORN CAKE	35
ORANGE LOAF CAKE	37
ZUCCHINI CHEESE BREAD – NO YEAST	39
MOIST BANANA CHOCOLATE LOAF	41
ESPRESSO AND DATE LOAF	43
LEMON CAKE	45

CHEESECAKES

NO BAKE MANGO CHEESECAKE	49
NO BAKE PASSION FRUIT CHEESECAKE	51
NO BAKE BAILEY'S CHOCOLATE CHEESECAKE	53
FERRERO ROCHER COFFEE CHEESECAKE	55
NO BAKE BLACKFOREST CHEESECAKE	57
NO BAKE LIME CHEESECAKE	59
NO BAKE MINT CHEESECAKE	61

CUPCAKES

- RICH BLACK FOREST CUPCAKES ... 65
- STRAWBERRY CREAM CHEESE CUPCAKES ... 67
- CARROT CUPCAKES ... 69
- CHOCOLATE GANACHE CUPCAKES ... 71
- LEMON CUPCAKES ... 73
- MOCHA CUPCAKES ... 75
- PINEAPPLE CUPCAKES ... 77
- LAVENDER CUPCAKES ... 79
- CHANTILLY DREAM CUPCAKES WITH RASPBERRY COMPOTE ... 83
- CHANTILLY EASTER BITES ... 85
- MATCHA GREEN TEA CUPCAKES ... 87
- BANANA LOVE IN EVERY BITE ... 89
- PISTACHIO WHITE CHOCOLATE CUPCAKES ... 91
- CREAMY, DREAMY IRISH DELIGHTS ... 93

OTHER

- SAVOURY MUFFINS ... 97
- APPLE PIE ... 99
- CARAMEL SLICE ... 101
- SUNSHINE IN A SQUARE ... 103
- BROWNIES ... 105
- EGGLESS CHOCOLATE PANCAKES ... 107
- THE BEST LEMON CURD ... 108
- TWO INGREDIENTS CHOCOLATE GANACHE ... 109
- WHITE CHOCOLATE GANACHE ... 110
- CHOCOLATE SHARDS ... 110
- STRAWBERRY COMPOTE ... 111
- BUTTER CREAM ... 112
- ITALIAN BUTTER CREAM ... 112
- FRESH CREAM FROSTING ... 113
- CREAM CHEESE DIP ... 114
- LEMON BUTTER CREAM ... 115

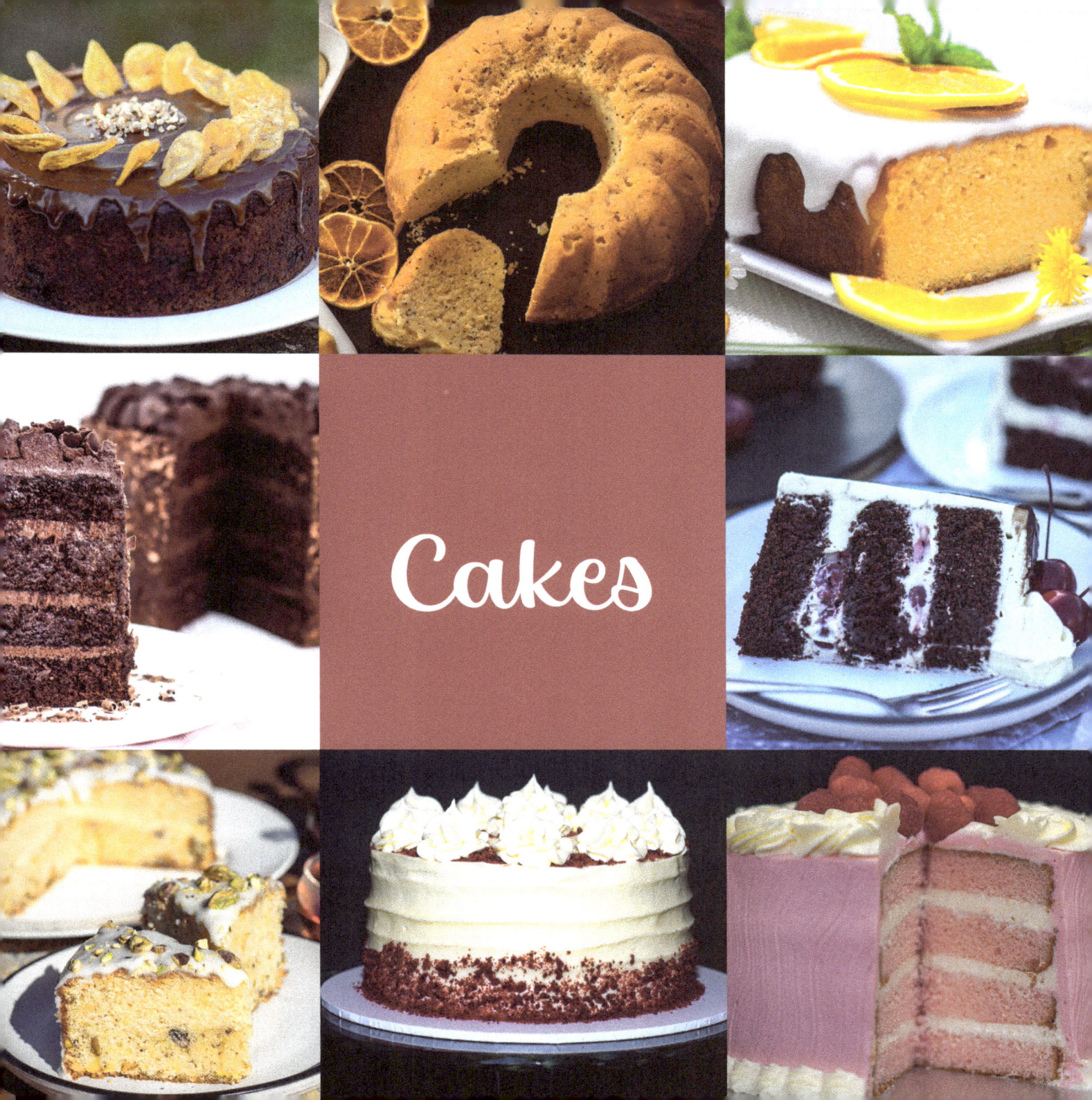

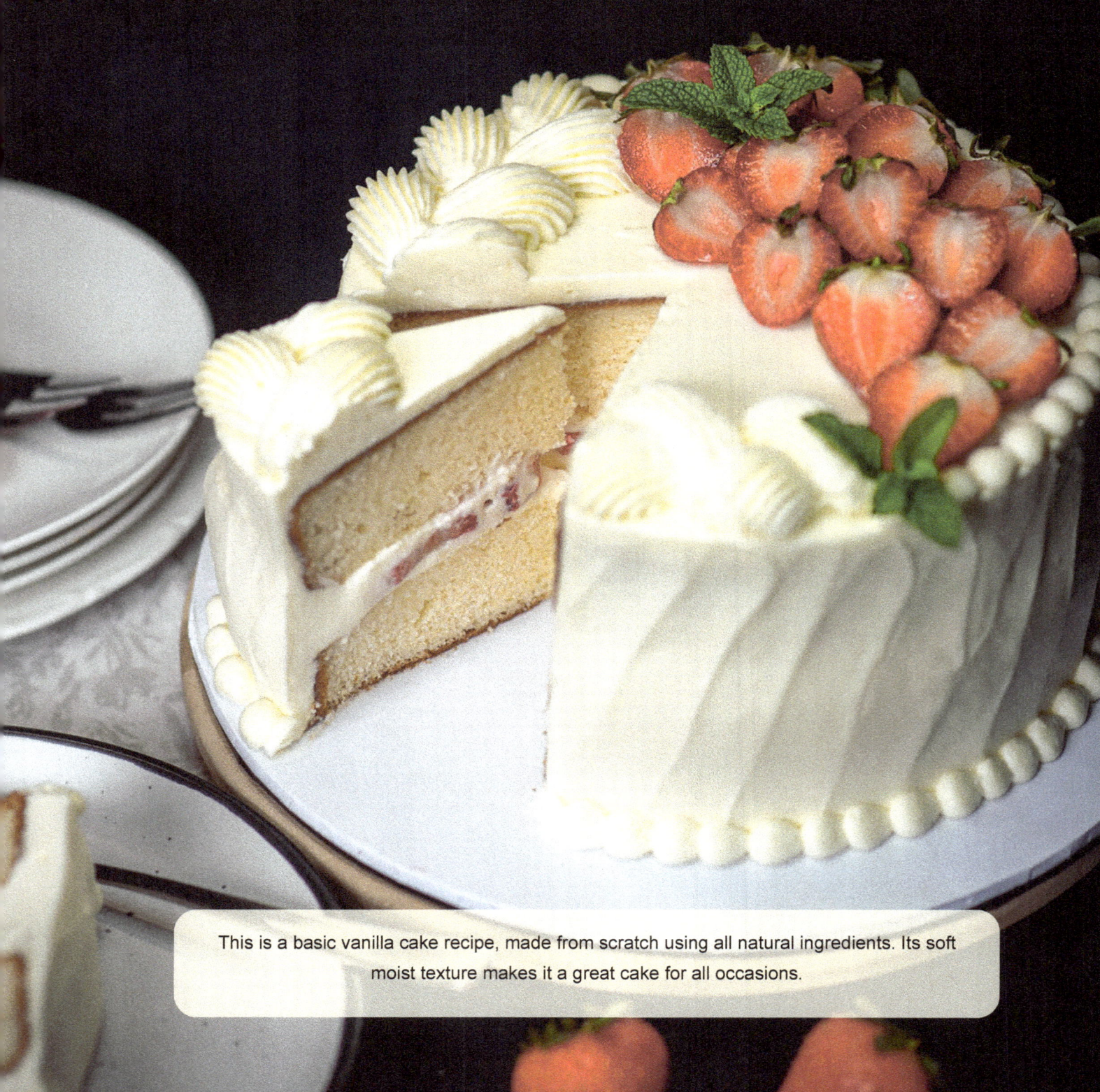

This is a basic vanilla cake recipe, made from scratch using all natural ingredients. Its soft moist texture makes it a great cake for all occasions.

MOIST VANILLA GOODNESS

Ingredients

225g (1 cup) unsalted butter - *softened*

330g (1½ cups) caster sugar

4 large eggs - *room temperature*

1 tbsp vanilla extract

375g (2½ cups) plain flour

2½ tsp baking powder

½ tsp salt

250ml (1 cup) whole milk - *room temperature*

Frosting

625 ml (2½ cups) thickened cream.

160g (1 cup) powdered sugar

1 tsp vanilla extract

450g (16oz) mascarpone cheese - *cold*

Garnish

3 cups strawberries

Method

1. Preheat oven to 160 °C fan forced. Lightly grease the sides and bottom of two 8" round cake tins. Line the bottoms with parchment paper. Generously grease the parchment paper. Dust the pans with flour then tap out any excess, set aside.
2. In a large bowl, beat butter and sugar together until light and fluffy - about 5 minutes. Add the eggs one at time, mixing well after each addition. Beat in vanilla.
3. In a medium bowl combine the flour, baking powder, and salt. Stir and whisk, then add it to the butter mixture. Finally add milk and beat on medium-low speed just until combined.
4. Divide the batter evenly between the two prepared tins.
5. Bake for 40 minutes, or until a skewer inserted into a centre comes out with a few moist crumbs attached. Take care not to over bake.
6. Cool for 10 minutes. Remove from tins and cool completely on a wire rack.

Making the frosting

7. Place mixing bowl and whisk attachment in the freezer for about 5 to 10 minutes to chill.
8. Spoon the cold mascarpone and thickened cream into a bowl and beat on medium speed, while slowly pouring the thickened cream, allowing the mascarpone cheese turn to a liquid consistency.
9. Add the powdered sugar and vanilla extract, increasing the mixing speed to high. Beat until soft peaks form.

Assembly

10. Place one layer on a serving plate. Put half of the frosting into a large piping bag, fitted with a large open round tip. Pipe a thick border around the edge of the cake. Add on fresh strawberries.
11. Pipe another thin layer of frosting over the strawberries and spread evenly with a spatula.
12. Place the second layer of cake on top. Frost the top and sides using a spatula. Once the cake is covered, remove the excess frosting using an icing smoother.
13. Use the remaining frosting to pipe florets on top using a large open star tip
14. Garnish with the leftover strawberries.
15. The cake should then be refrigerated.

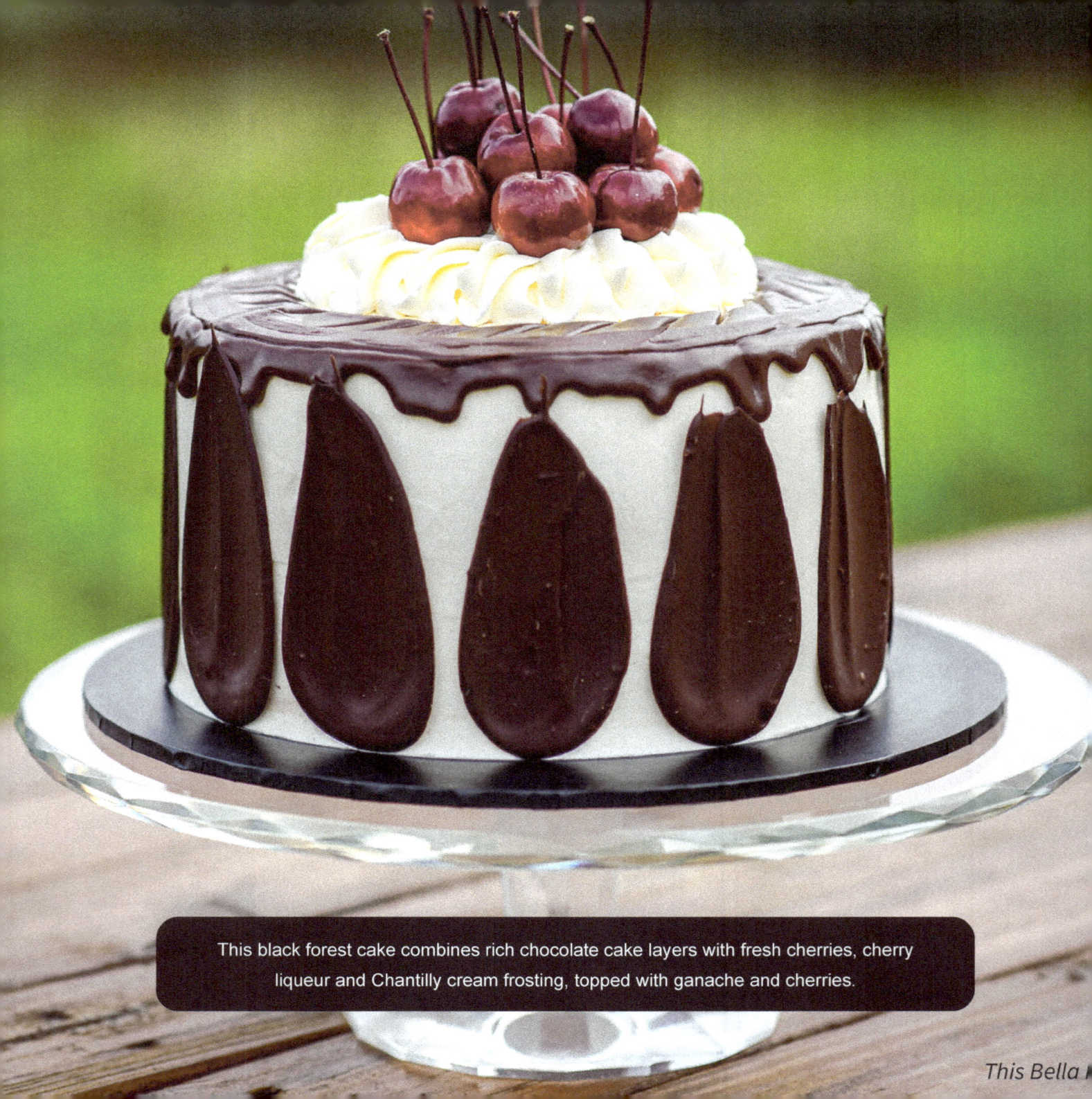

This black forest cake combines rich chocolate cake layers with fresh cherries, cherry liqueur and Chantilly cream frosting, topped with ganache and cherries.

RICH BLACKFOREST CAKE

Ingredients

Chocolate Cake

263g (1¾ cups) all-purpose flour
330g (1½ cups) sugar
75g (¾ cup) Dutch cocoa powder
1 ½ tsp baking powder
1 ½ tsp baking soda
½ tsp salt
3 large eggs - *at room temperature*
2 tsp vanilla extract
250ml (1 cup) milk
120ml (½ cup) vegetable oil
50 ml espresso
250ml (1 cup) boiling water

Cherry filling

500g morello cherries in syrup
1 tsp lemon juice
½ tbsp corn flour
110g (½ cup) caster sugar
118ml (½ cup) any liqueur Kirsch, brandy or spice rum)

Chantilly Cream

750ml (3 cups) thickened cream
2 tsp vanilla
7 tbsp powdered sugar
2 tbsp milk powder

For Decorating

100g dark chocolate - 70 %
Fresh cherries

Method

Chocolate Cake

1. Preheat oven to 160°C fan forced. Grease two baking 8" tins with butter. Line with parchment/ baking paper
2. In a small bowl sift flour, cocoa powder, baking powder, baking soda, sugar and salt set aside
3. In mixing bowl beat eggs, oil, vanilla extract, milk and add espresso
4. Add the dry ingredients to the egg mixture, being careful not to over mix
5. Continue adding the hot water until just combined.
6. Pour the batter into the prepared tins - the batter should be pourable
7. Bake for 45 minutes, or until the skewer inserted into the cake centre comes out clean
8. Allow to cool in the tins for 10 minutes before turning the cakes out onto a rack to completely cool.

Cherry Filling

9. Drain off the syrup from the cherries. Heat the syrup in a pan on medium heat, add the sugar bringing to a gentle simmer. Then stir in corn slurry and add lemon juice. Remove from the heat and stir in the liquor. Pour to drain cherries. Allow to completely cool

Chantilly Cream

10. In the large mixing bowl add whipped cream, sugar, milk powder, vanilla and whisk with electric mixer for 3 -5 minutes until stiff peaks

Let's Decorate

11. Add first layer of cake to a serving plate. Brush with the cherry liquid and add a ¼ cup of Chantilly cream.

12. Fit the end of piping bag with open star piping tip and pipe a tube of frosting around the top of the cream.

13. Add half of the cherry mixture and spread evenly with spatula or spoon.

14. Add the next layer of cake and repeat until all cake layers are on.

15. For the top of the cake, repeat this process. Adding the chocolate ganache instead of cherry filling.

16. Spread the cream evenly around the side and stick the chocolate shards over the cream all around cake

17. To finish, pipe swirls of the cream on top of the cake and garnish with cherries.

Notes

For Chocolate Shards recipe see page 110
For Chocolate ganache recipe see page 109

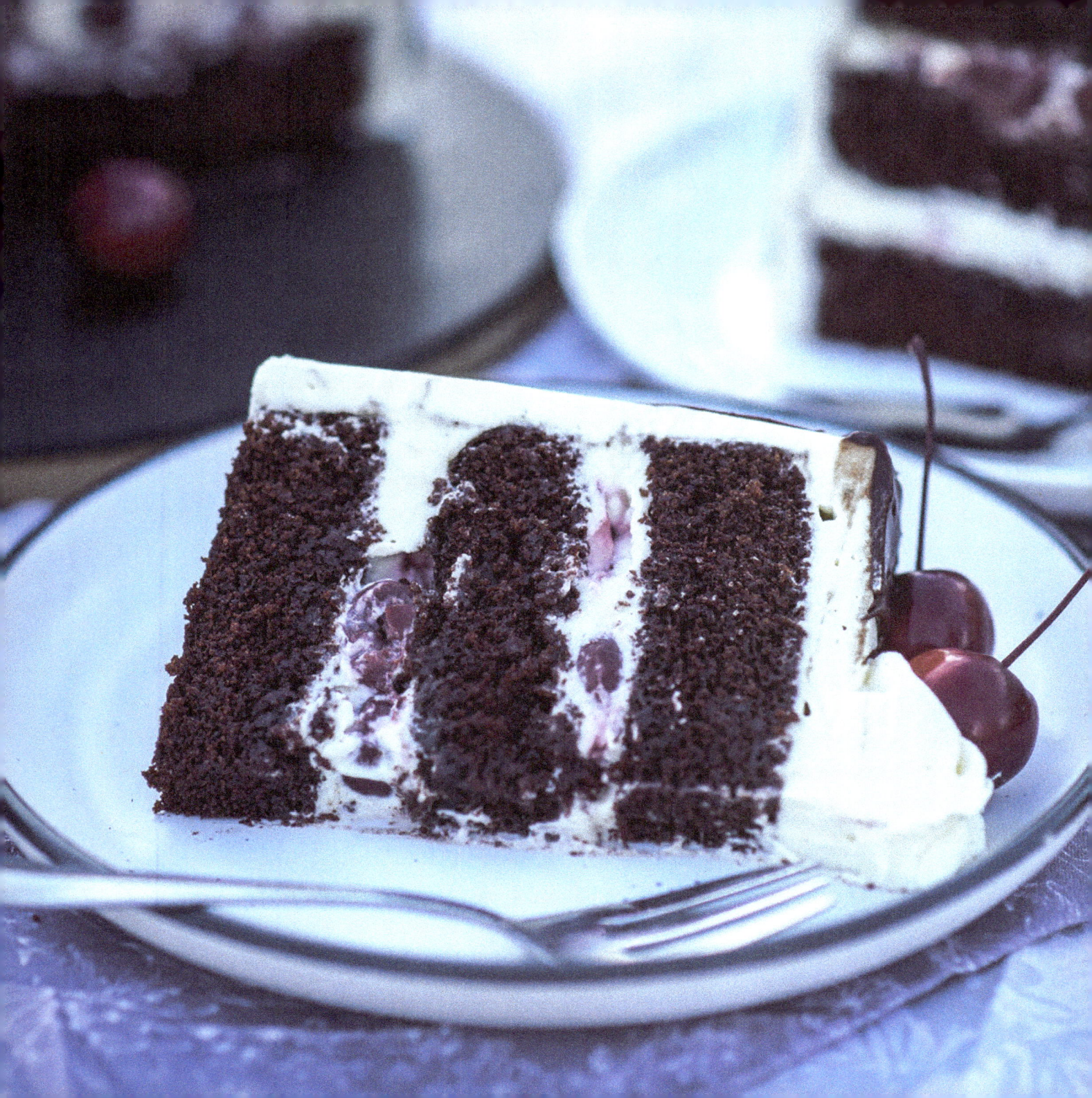

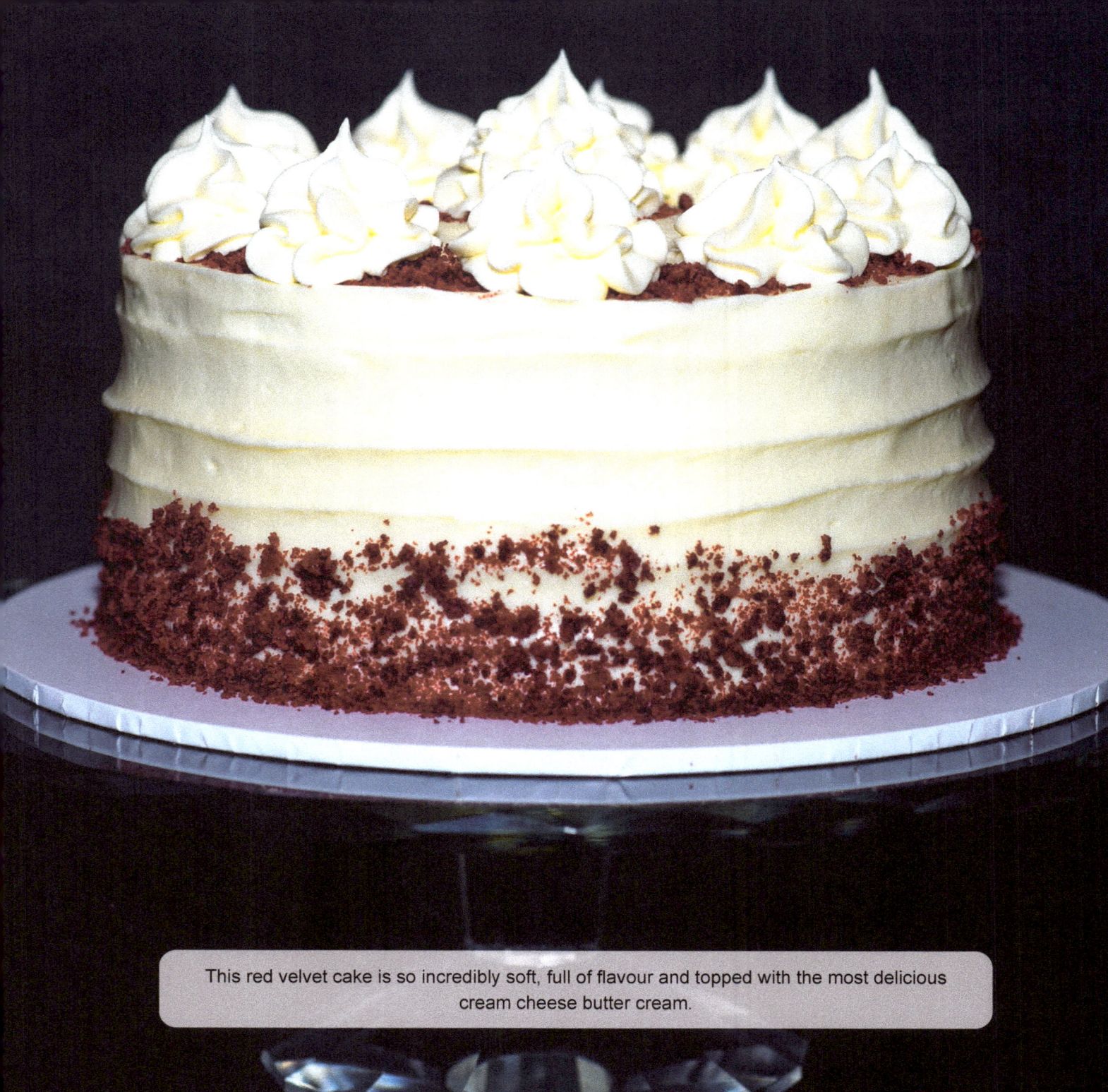

This red velvet cake is so incredibly soft, full of flavour and topped with the most delicious cream cheese butter cream.

RED VELVET PERFECTION

Ingredients

235g (1 1/2 cup + 1 tbsp) plain flour

18g corn flour

14g cocoa powder - *unsweetened*

1 tsp baking powder

½ tsp baking soda

½ tsp salt

113g (approx. ½ cup) unsalted butter – *room temperature*

180ml (¾ cup) vegetable oil

330g (approx. 1½ cups) granulated white sugar

3 large eggs - room temperature

1 tbsp vanilla extract

1 ½ tsp white vinegar

165ml (⅔ cup) milk - *room temperature*

2 tsp red food colouring - *gel or liquid*

Cream cheese frosting

452g full fat cream cheese - *softened to room temperature*

150g (approx. ⅔ cup) unsalted butter - *softened to room temperature*

400g (2½ cups) soft icing sugar

½ tsp vanilla extract

Method

1. Preheat oven to 160 °C fan forced. Grease two 8" cake tins and line with baking paper.

2. Sift flour, corn flour, cocoa powder, baking soda, baking powder and salt in a bowl. Set aside

3. Add butter, sugar and vegetable oil in another bowl. Using an electric mixer cream together for 2-3 minutes until light and fluffy. Add eggs, one by one while mixing well. Add vanilla, red food colour and vinegar. Mix well until combined.

4. Mix in half of the premixed dry ingredients to the wet mixture, alternating with milk and gently fold with spatula until just combined. Add the remaining dry ingredients and gently fold it into the mixture until just combined. Do not over mix.

5. Transfer the batter evenly into the 2 x 8-inch cake tins, and bake for 45 minutes, or until the skewer comes

out clean. Be careful not to open the oven door too early; it can cause the cake to sink.

6. Once baked, allow to cool for 15 minutes, and then turn cakes out onto a wire rack before frosting with cream cheese.

Making the frosting

7. Add cream cheese and butter to a large bowl and beat together on medium to high speed until smooth (use a handheld mixer, or stand mixer fitted with a paddle attachment) Add soft icing sugar, vanilla extract and a pinch of salt. Beat on low speed for 30 seconds and increase to high speed for about 3 minutes until completely combined and creamy. Frosting should be soft but not runny.

Assembly

8. Using a knife, slice a thin layer off the top of the cakes to create a flat surface. Discard or crumble over the finished cake. Place 1 cake layer on a cake stand or serving plate. Cover the top evenly with frosting. Top with the 2nd layer and spread remaining frosting over the top and sides. Use an open star piping tip for the topper.

9. Refrigerate for an hour before slicing to help the cake hold its shape when cutting.

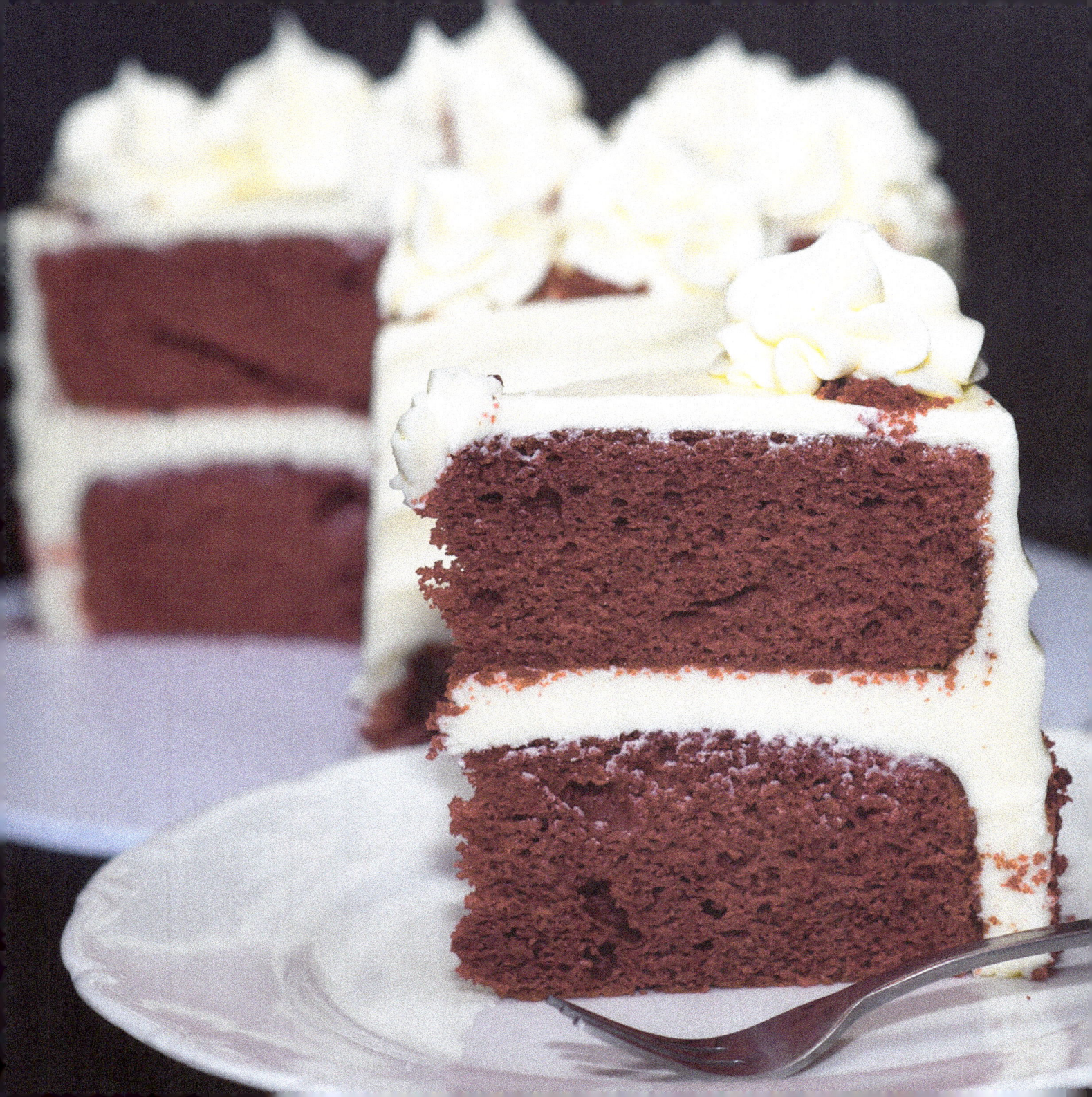

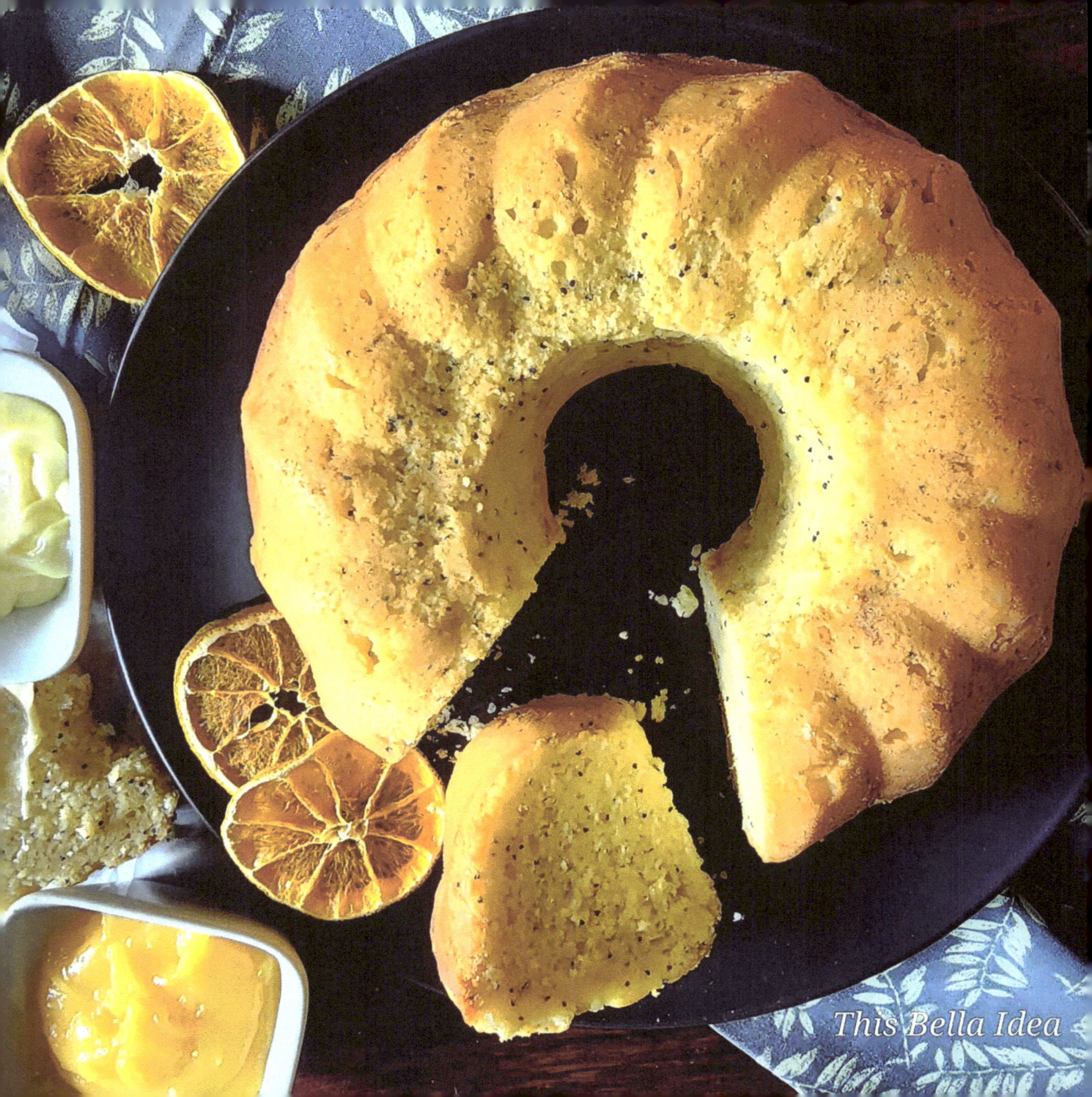

LEMON AND POPPY SEED TREATS

This continental-style cake is very easy to make resulting in a delicious, pleasant tasting, "all-purpose" cake. It matches perfectly with morning or afternoon tea. Can be served with cream cheese or lemon curd.

Ingredients

150g (⅔ cup) unsalted butter - *softened*
145g (⅔ cup) caster sugar
3 large eggs - *lightly beaten - room temperature*
2 lemons - *finely grated zest and juice*
1 tbsp Greek yogurt - *room temperature*
1 tsp vanilla extract
125ml (½ cup) milk - *room temperature*
300g (2 cups) plain flour
1 tbsp poppy seeds
1 tsp baking powder
¼ tsp of salt

Method

1. Preheat oven to 160 °C fan-forced. Lightly grease a bundt tin 23 cm (9 inch) generously with butter and dust with flour.

2. Put the butter and caster sugar into a large bowl and, using a hand mixer or electric mixer, cream together until pale and fluffy. Gradually beat in the eggs, one at a time mixing constantly, followed by the lemon zest and juice, yogurt, vanilla extract, milk and poppy seeds.

3. Sift the flour, baking powder and salt into the bowl, then use a large metal spoon or spatula to fold it in. Spoon the mixture into the prepared tin.

4. Bake for about 40 minutes or until a skewer inserted into the centre comes out clean. Leave to cool in the tin, and then turn out onto a wire rack. When the cake is cold, transfer to a cake stand or serving plate.

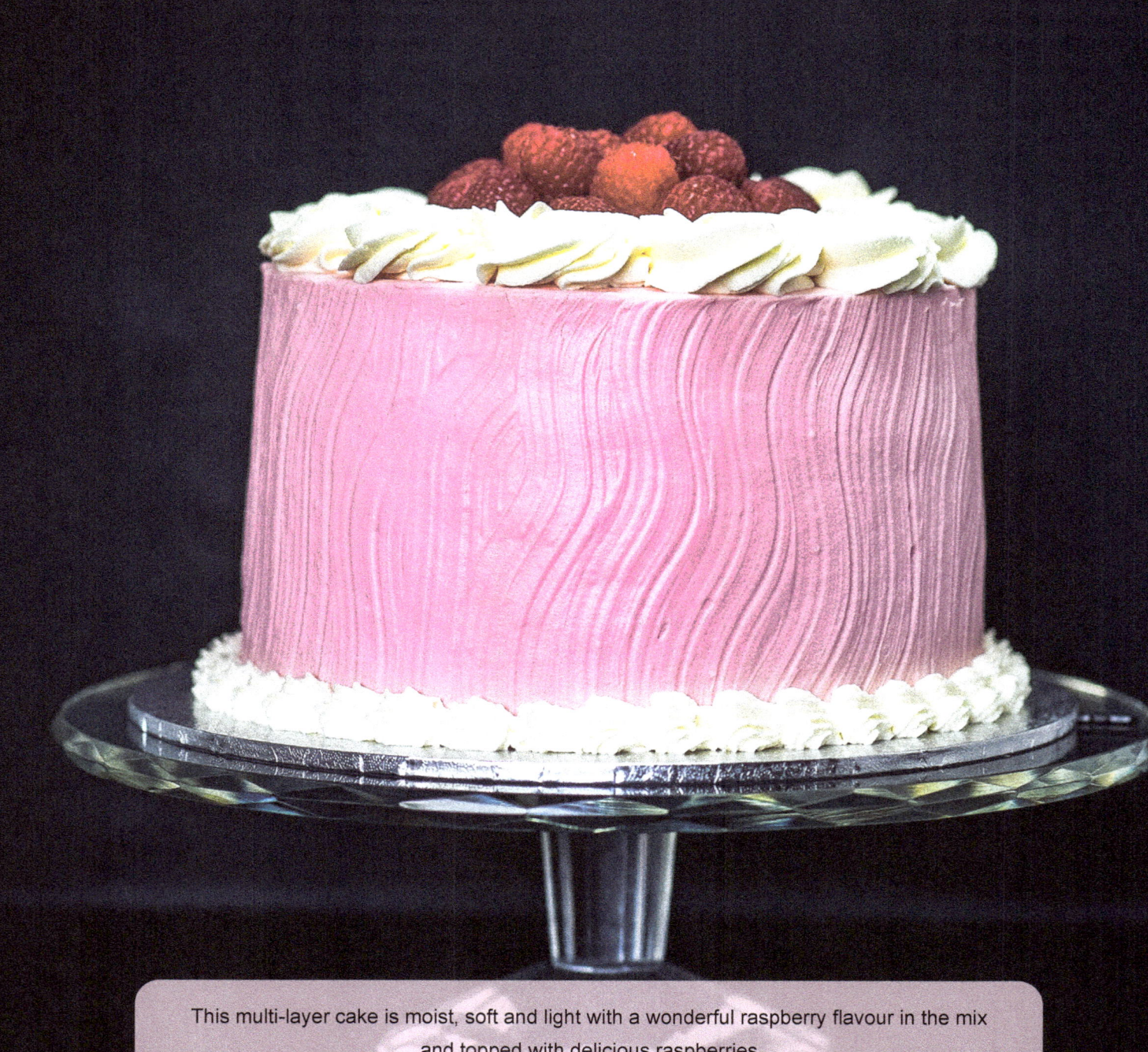
This multi-layer cake is moist, soft and light with a wonderful raspberry flavour in the mix and topped with delicious raspberries

RASPBERRY CAKE WITH WHITE CHOCOLATE GANACHE

Ingredients

170g (¾ cup) unsalted butter - *room temperature*

440g (2 cups) sugar

3 large eggs - *room temperature*

450g (3 cups) plain flour

2 tsp baking powder

½ tsp baking soda

¼ tsp salt

250ml (1 cup) sour cream

60ml (¼ cup) vegetable oil

1 tsp raspberry essence

Pink colour gel - *just use a small amount to brighten up the colour*

White Chocolate Ganache

210g white chocolate or white chocolate chips - *finely chopped*

83g (⅓ cup) thickened cream

For making fresh cream frosting see page 113

For making butter cream frosting see page 112

Method

Making the white chocolate ganache

1. The ganache filling needs about 3 hours to set, so I recommend making it first.. Place 210g of white chocolate in a medium size bowl and set aside.
2. Pour the thickened cream into a heat proof bowl and heat in 15 second intervals in
3. microwave until it just begins to bubble.
4. Pour the thickened cream over the white chocolate, let the mixture sit for a couple of minutes.
5. Use a spatula to mix the ganache mixture until it has blended together and smooth. Press some plastic wrap against the ganache and place the bowl in the fridge to chill.

Making the raspberry cake

1. Preheat oven to 160 °C fan forced. Grease three 8" round cake tins and line with parchment paper.
2. In a medium sized bowl, add flour, baking powder, baking soda and salt, whisk until combined.
3. In another bowl, combined the sour cream, oil and raspberry flavour. Blend with fork and set aside.
4. Use a mixer to mix the butter until smooth, gradually add the sugar and mix on medium speed for 3 to 5 minutes until pale and fluffy.
5. Add the eggs one at a time, mix well.
6. Add the flour mixture and the sour cream mixture.
7. Add the pink colouring gel, mix until combined and smooth. Do not over mix.
8. Bake at 160 C for 40-45 minutes or until the skewer inserted into the centre comes out clean.
9. Let it cool in tins and turn out to cooling rack.
10. Using a large, serrated edge knife, remove the domes from the top, so the cake layers are flat and level.
11. Place the first cake on a serving platter. Spread half a cup of butter cream, or fresh cream evenly over the top of the cake, then use the frosting to create a dam wall around the outer edge. Spread about half of the white chocolate ganache into an even layer inside of the wall, then level out the wall and the ganache so that it's all evenly layered.
12. Continue layering by adding another layer of cake on top of the ganache, then repeat the process until the final layer for top cake.
13. Use an offset spatula to frost the top and outside of the cake layer and pipe swirl around the outer edge of the cake. Top each swirl with fresh raspberry if you like.

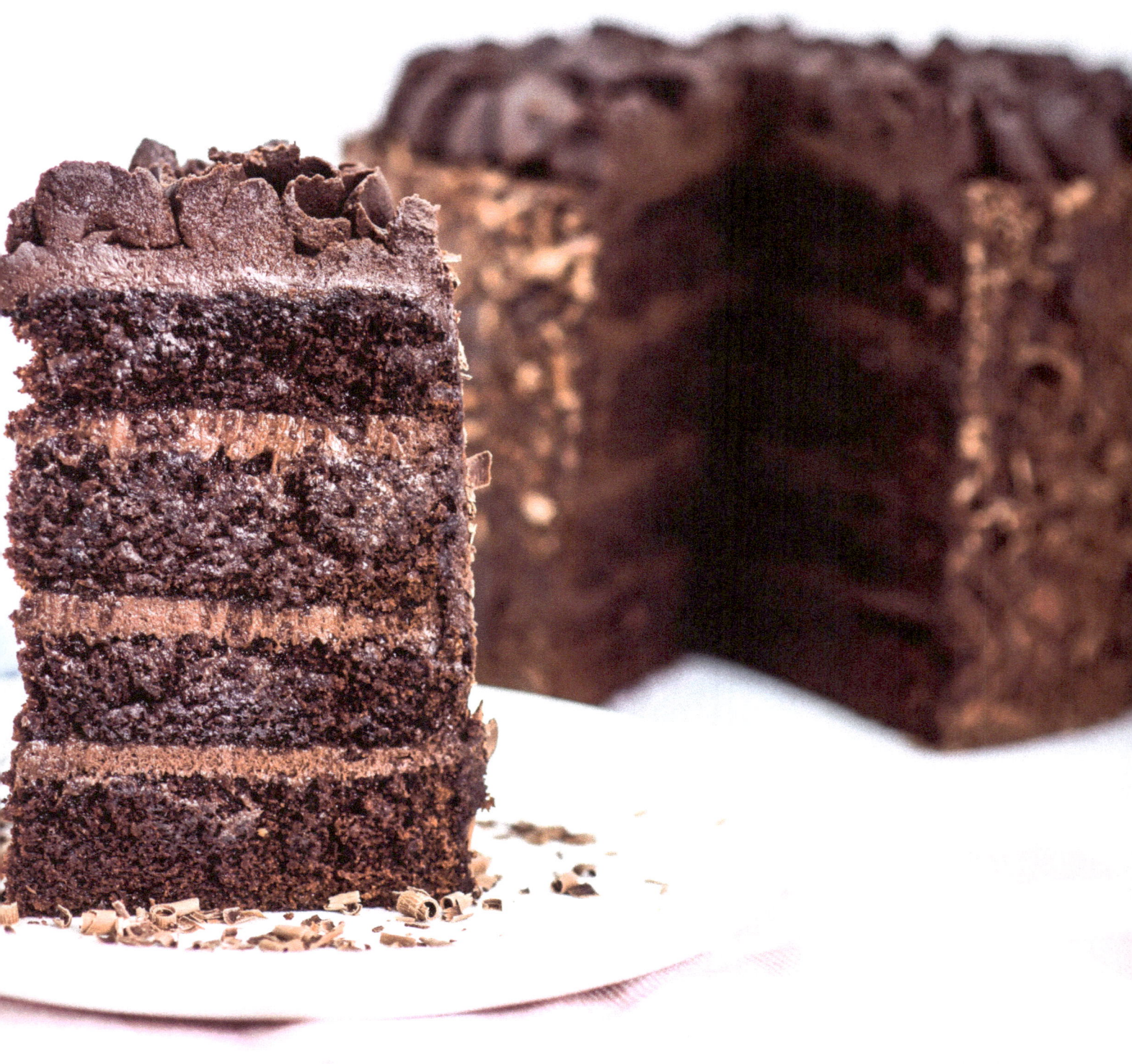

CHOCOLATE GANACHE CAKE

Ingredients

300g (2 cups) all-purpose flour
440g (2 cups) granulated sugar
75g (¾ cups) cocoa powder
2 tsp baking powder
1½ tsp baking soda
1 tsp salt
2 tbsp espresso powder
250ml (1 cup milk) - *at room temperature*
3 eggs- *at room temperature*
2 tsp vanilla extract
115ml (½ cup) vegetable oil
250ml (1 cup) boiling water

For the chocolate ganache

250ml (1 cup) thickened cream
198g (7/8 cup) unsalted butter - *- at room temperature; chopped*
428g (2¼ cups) dark chocolate chips - *at least 60% of cocoa solids*

Method

1. Preheat oven to 170 °C fan forced. Grease and line 4 x 7-inch round cake tins
2. In a medium bowl, whisk together flour, sugar, cocoa powder, baking powder, salt and espresso powder.
3. In a large mixing bowl, whisk together milk, eggs, vanilla extract and oil
4. Gradually add the dry ingredients to the wet ingredients and mix. Reduce the speed and carefully add the boiling water. The mixture will be very runny. And that's exactly what we want.
5. Divide the batter evenly among the prepared tins and smooth the top
6. Bake for 35 – 40 minutes our until skewer comes out clean. Let the cakes cool in the pan for about 10 minutes before transferring them to a wire rack to cool completely

The chocolate ganache

7. Heat the thickened cream in a small saucepan over a medium heat until it starts to simmer
8. Remove from the heat and pour over the chopped butter and chocolate chips in a heatproof bowl. Let it set for 3 minutes, before stirring until smooth and glossy.

Assembly

9. Once the cake is completely cool, place one layer on the serving plate, and spread a layer of ganache on the top. Place the next cake layer on top and repeat the process for the second and third cake layers
10. Frost the outside of the cake, with the remaining ganache and decorate as desired.

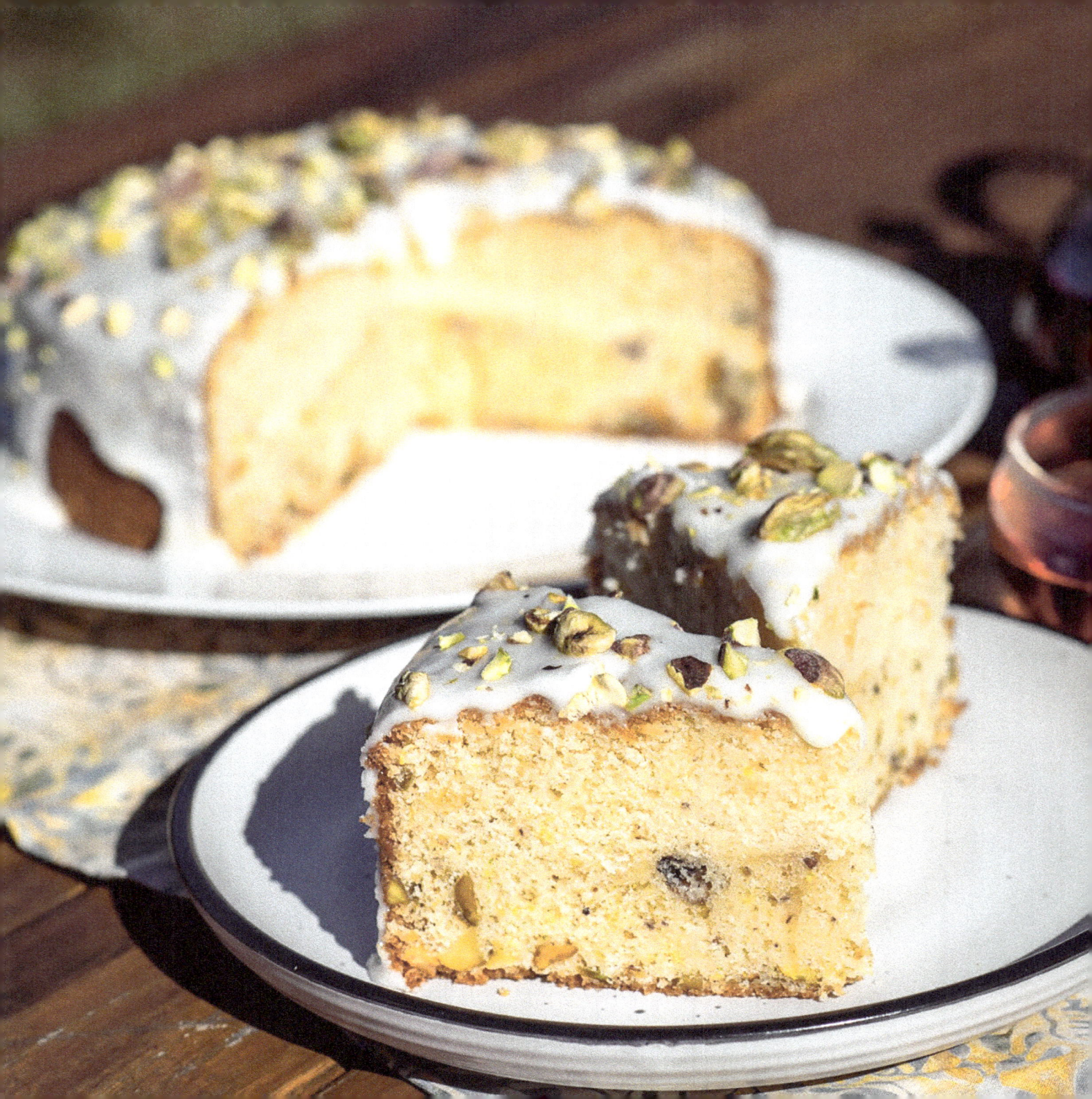

PISTACHIO CAKE WITH A LEMON KISS

The delightful crunch of pistachios combines together perfectly with lemon in this rich butter cake.

Ingredients

40g pistachio kernels - *chopped*
3 eggs
220g (1 cup) white sugar - *granulated*
150g (1 cup) self-raising flour
125ml (½ cup) milk - *at room temperature*
1 tbsp finely grated orange zest
113g (½ cup) salted butter - *melted*
125g pistachio kernels - *roughly chopped*

The glaze
240g (1½ cup) icing sugar
1 tsp finely grated lemon zest
3 tsp lemon juice

Method

1. Preheat oven to 160 °C fan forced. Grease a 9" round cake tin and line base with baking paper.

2. Using a hand held beater or stand mixer, beat all the cake ingredients, except the self-raising flour and pistachio, for 2 minutes. Gently fold in self-raising flour and pistachios.

3. Spoon the cake batter evenly into the tin

4. Bake for 40-50 minutes, or until the metal skewer inserted into the centre comes out clean.

5. Leave to stand in the tin for 5 minutes before turning out onto a wire rack to cool completely.

Making the glaze

6. Mix together the icing sugar, orange zest and stir in the lemon juice to make it a pouring consistency

7. Spoon the glaze over the cooled cake and sprinkle with the pistachios.

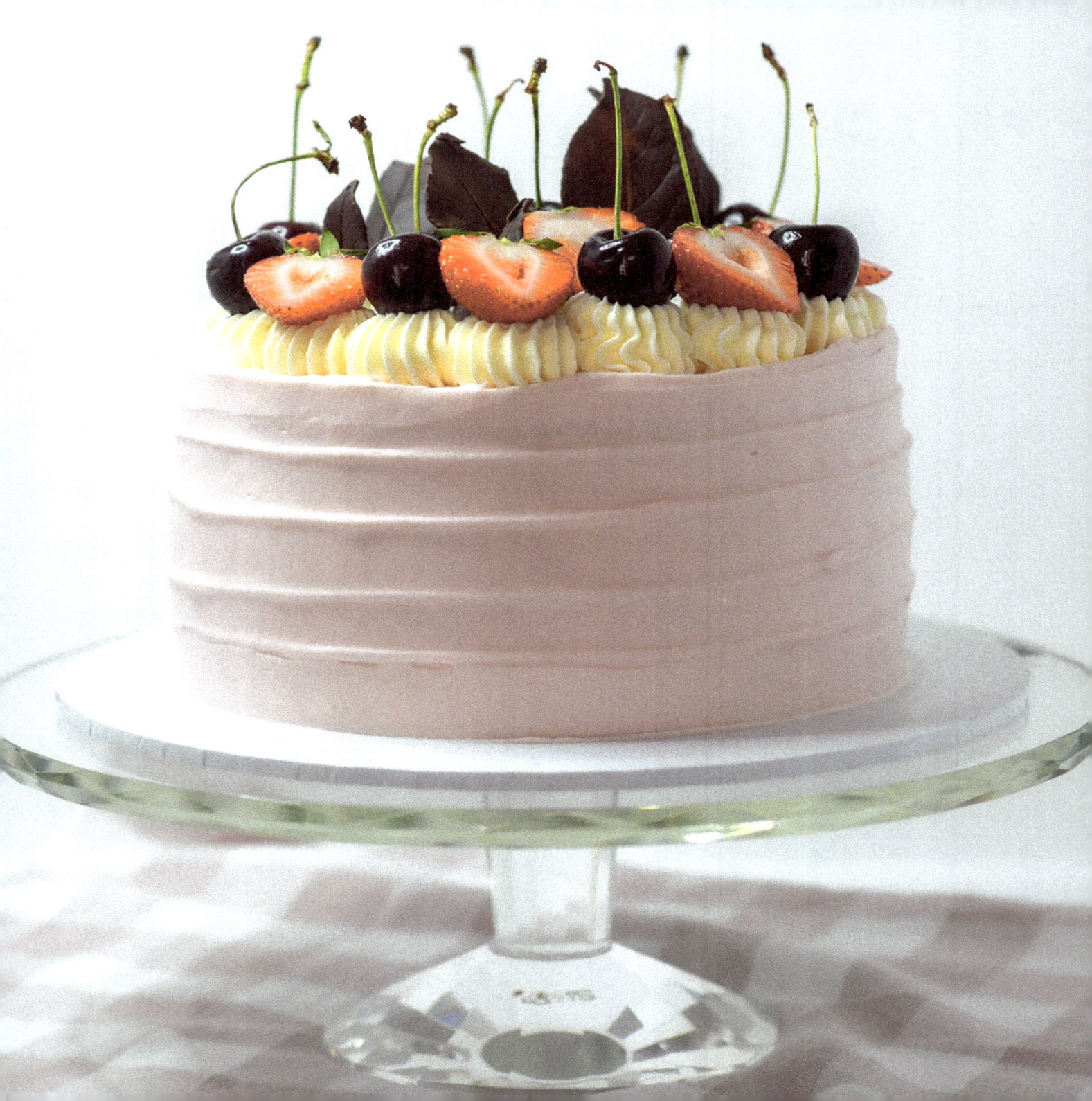

BUTTER CAKE

This classic tea cake is quick and easy to make and perfect for any occasion. Add frosting with simple butter cream and one slice will never be enough.

Ingredients

113g (½ cup) unsalted butter - *at room temperature*
145g (⅔ cup) caster sugar
2 tsp vanilla
3 large eggs - *at room temperature*
263g (1 ¾ cups) flour
2 ½ tsp baking powder
¼ tsp salt
188ml (¾ cup) milk

For the frosting

113g (½ cup) unsalted butter - *at room temperature*
320g (2 cups) soft icing sugar - *sifted*
1 tsp vanilla
2 tbsp thickened cream - *at room temperature*
A few drops of pink food gel - *optional*

For garnish

Fresh strawberry or fresh cherries

Method

1. Preheat oven to 160 °C fan forced. Grease and line an 8" round cake tins with baking paper
2. In a large mixing bowl, mix butter, sugar and vanilla until pale and creamy. Then add eggs one at the time. Beat until well combined
3. In a separate bowl, whisk flour, baking powder and salt.
4. Add half of the flour mixture, to the butter mixture, along with the milk and mix on low speed. Add the remaining flour mixture and continue to mix until the cake batter is smooth and creamy.
5. Pour cake batter into the prepared cake tin and bake in the oven for 40-45 minutes or until skewer inserted into middle of the cake comes out clean.

The Frosting

6. Mix the butter until creamy and smooth. Add vanilla, sugar and thickened cream. Continue to beat until smooth and fluffy. If desired add the food gel colouring and mix until frosting changes colour.
7. Spread the frosting on top and the sides of the cake, and use the piping tip for decoration
8. Top with fresh fruit as desired

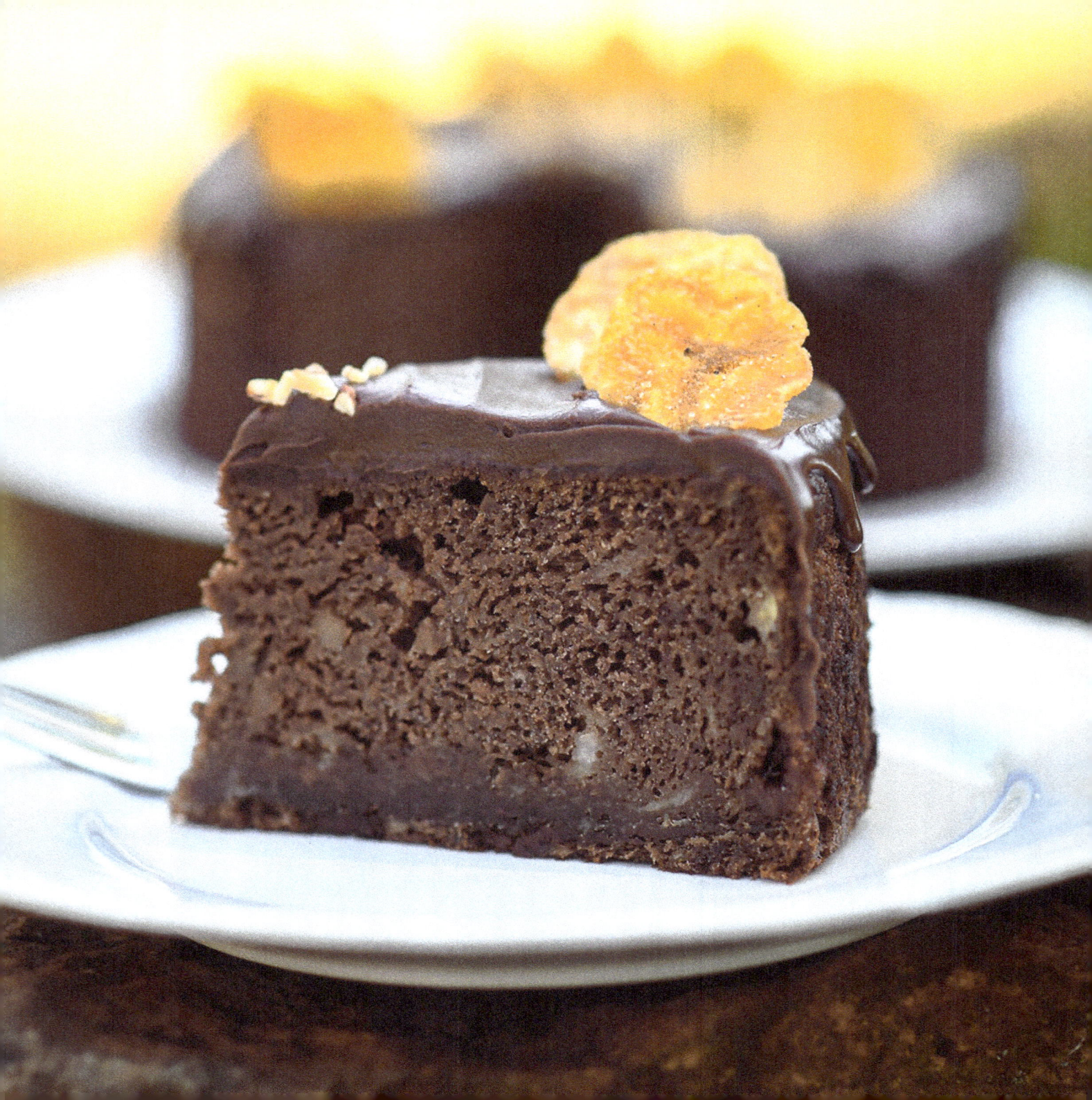

BANANA CHOCOLATE CAKE

This delicious cake is quite moist and fudgy. Suitable for any occasion and best served on the second day after baking.

Ingredients

170g (¾ cup) unsalted butter - *at room temperature*

220g (1 cup) white sugar

110g (½ cup) brown sugar

2 eggs - *at room temperature*

1½ cup mashed banana (from 3 ripe bananas)

1 tsp vanilla

300g (2 cups) cake flour

75g (¾ cup) Dutch cocoa powder

1½ tsp baking powder

1 tsp baking soda

¾ tsp salt

¾ cup butter milk (1 tbsp vinegar + ¾ cup milk) - *at room temperature*

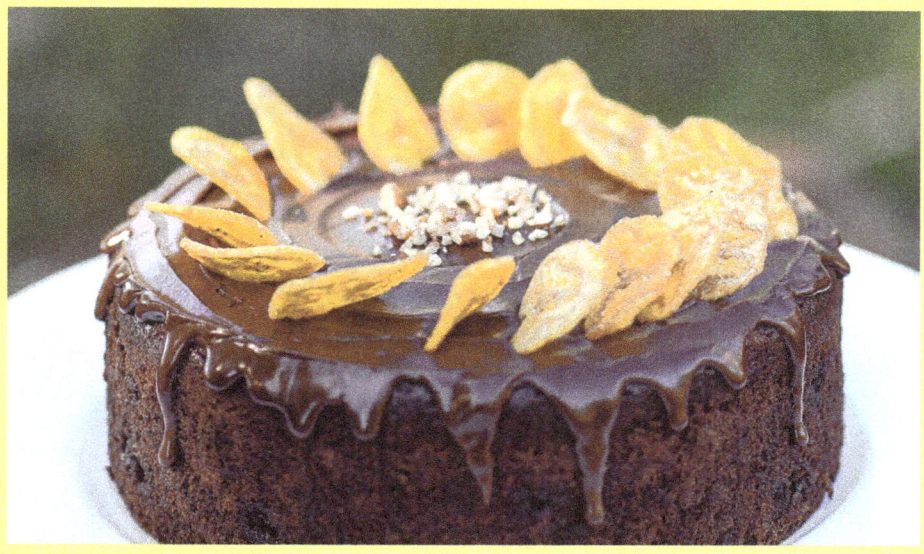

Method

1. Preheat oven to 170 °C fan forced. Grease an 8-inch round cake tin line with baking paper.
2. In a bowl, cream butter with the sugar and eggs – adding eggs one at a time
3. Mix mashed bananas with vanilla.
4. In a medium sized bowl sift flour, cocoa powder, baking powder, baking soda and salt.
5. Add flour mixture to butter mixture in 3 parts, then add butter milk.
6. Spread the mixture evenly into the cake tin and bake for 40-45 minutes or until skewer inserted to the cake comes clean.
7. Allow to completely cool and when cooled, frost generously with chocolate ganache and garnish with banana chips.

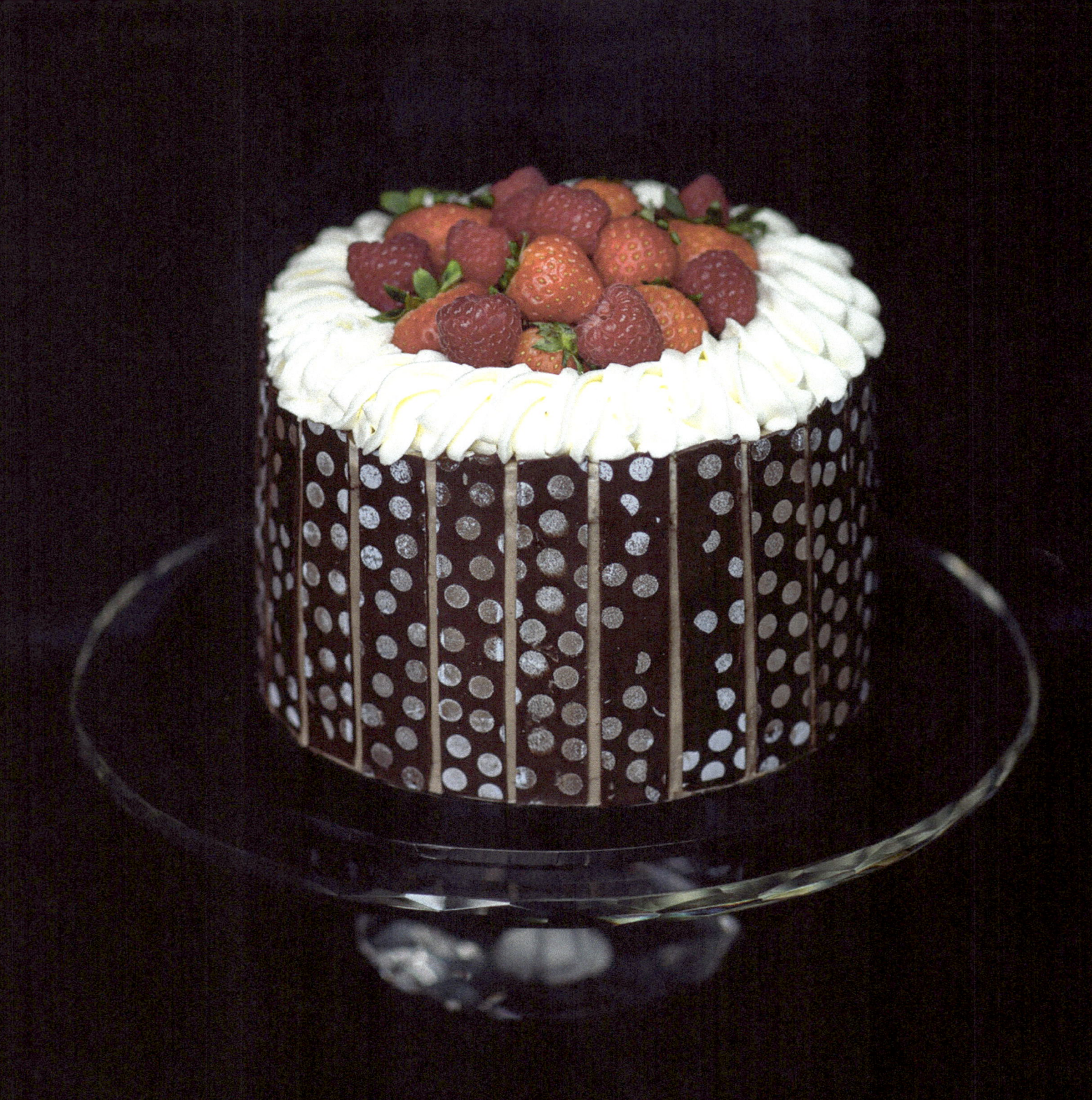

CHOCOLATE ESPRESSO CAKE

This cake is moist and rich - filled with two types of coffee to intensify the chocolate flavour.

Ingredients

300g (2 cups) all-purpose flour
50g (½ cup) Dutch cocoa powder
1½ tsp baking powder
225g (1 cup) unsalted butter
220g (1 cup) granulated sugar
110g (½ cup) brown sugar
3 eggs
1 tsp vanilla extract
1 cup brewed espresso coffee

Fresh Cream Frosting

375ml (1½ cups) thickened cream – *cold*
7 tbsp Powdered sugar – *sifted*
2 tbsp milk powder
1 tbsp vanilla

Garnish

Chocolate transfer sheet
Fresh strawberries

Method

1. Preheat oven to 170 °C fan forced.
2. In a medium bowl, combine the flour, cocoa powder, baking soda. Set aside
3. In a mixing bowl, combine the butter with sugars, eggs (one at the time) and vanilla extract. Mix until well combined
4. Slowly add the dry ingredients, folding in until incorporated
5. Pour in the brewed espresso and mix to combine with cake batter
6. Evenly divide the cake batter and pour into 2 lightly sprayed 8-inch cake pans. Gently tap on the counter to make sure all the air bubbles are settled
7. Bake for 45 minutes, until the cake springs back when touched. Remove from the oven and let them cool on the rack before frosting

The frosting

8. Place mixing bowl and whisk attachment in the freezer for 5 – 10 minutes to chill
9. Put the thickened cream in the mixing bowl and add powdered sugar, milk powder and vanilla. Beat at medium speed, increasing the speed to high. Beat until soft fluffy peaks form

Assembly

10. Place one cake layer on a cake stand or turntable and add ¾ of the frosting. Set the second cake layer on top and frost the top and sides of the whole cake until covered
11. Garnish with chocolate transfer sheet, piping the edges and add fresh strawberries

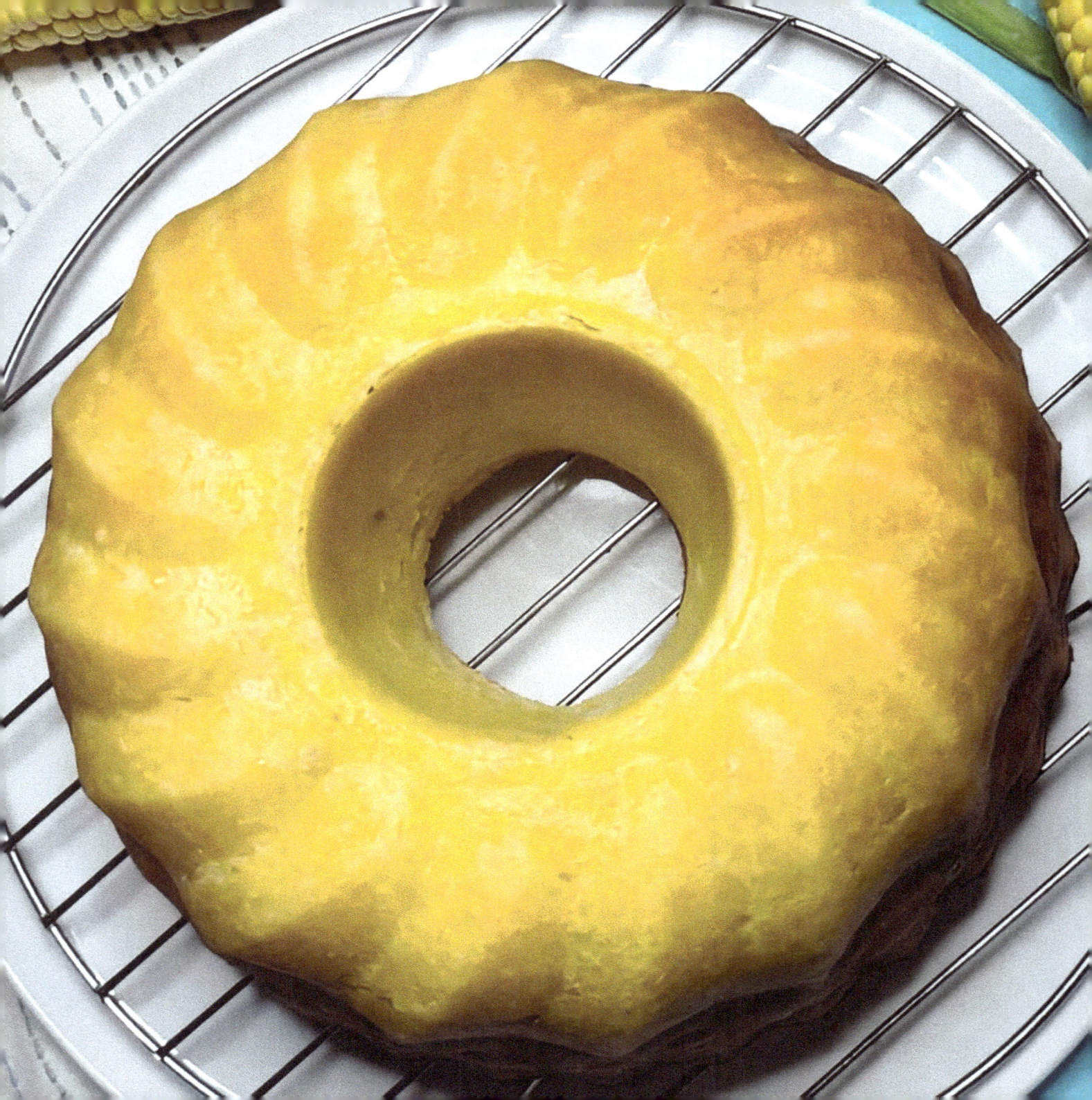

BRAZILIAN SWEET CORN CAKE

Easy to make and goes great with cup of tea or coffee.

Ingredients

2½ cups of fresh corn kernels (Approximately 4 cobs)
250ml (1 cup) whole milk
125 (½ cup) coconut milk
300g (2 cups) corn flour
330g (1½ cups) granulated sugar
175ml (¾ cup) vegetable oil
4 large eggs - *room temperature*
85g (1 cup) shredded coconut
1 tbsp baking powder
A pinch of salt

Method

1. Preheat oven to 170 °C fan forced. Butter and flour a 9" bundt cake tin
2. Combine the corn kernels and milk in a blender and blend until smooth.
3. Add coconut milk, cornflour, sugar, oil, eggs, coconut and salt. Pulse until well combined.
4. Add the baking powder and pulse twice, just to incorporate into the batter.
5. Put the batter into the prepared cake tin and bake for 50 minutes or until the skewer inserted in the centre comes out clean.
6. Remove from the oven and immediately run knife around the edges to loosen it. Let it cool completely about 20 minutes, then turn cake into a cooling rack.
7. Slice and serve… enjoy.

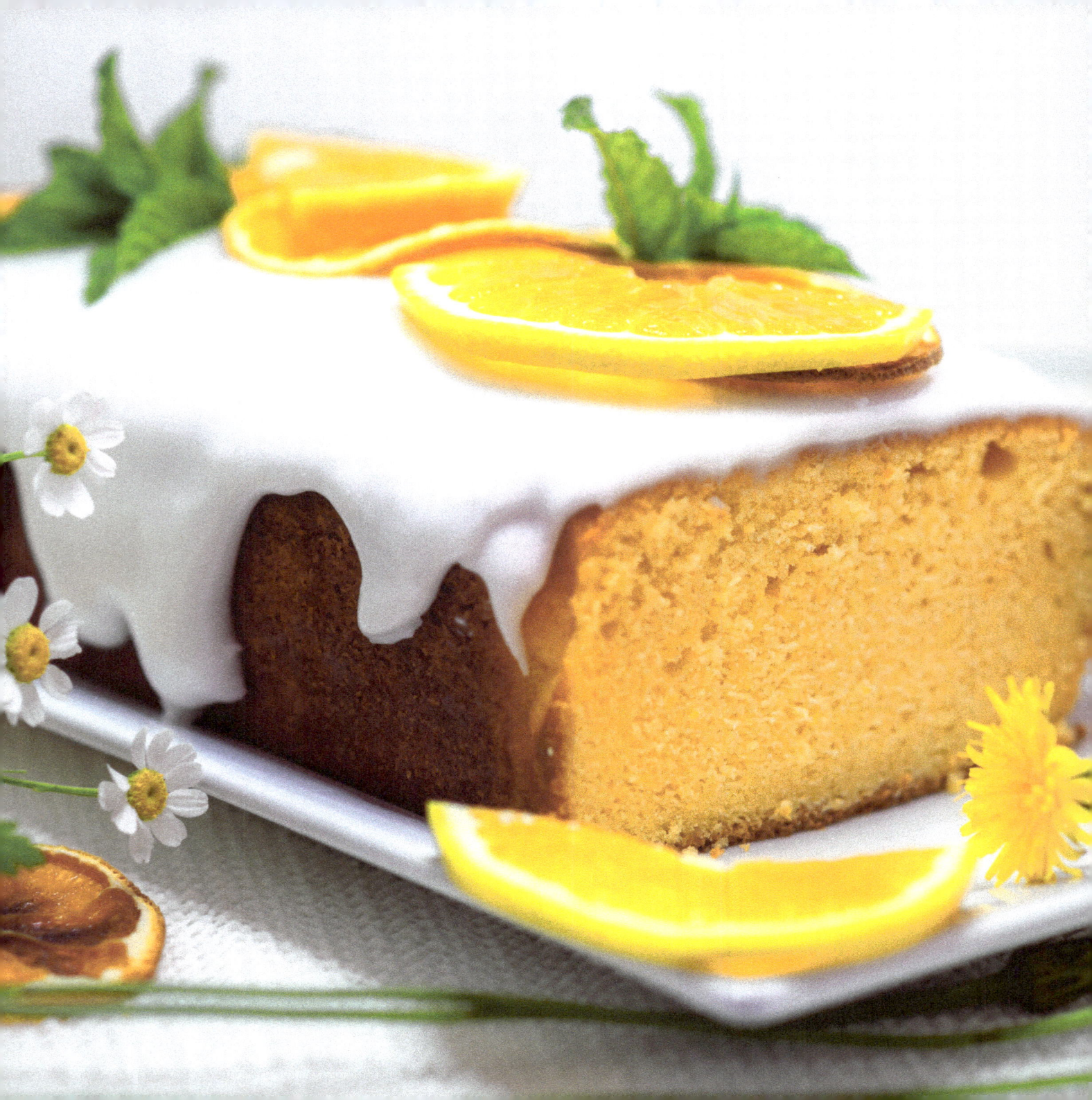

ORANGE LOAF CAKE

Oranges are cheap and readily available – two wonderful reasons why we should be cooking and baking with them. Combined with lemon icing glaze, this makes for the perfect cake to enjoy for morning tea, along with your favourite cup of tea or coffee.

Ingredients

113g (½ cup) butter- *at room temperature*
220g (1 cup) granulated sugar

2 large eggs - *at room temperature*
3 tbsp orange zest
120ml (½ cup) orange juice
300g (2 cups) cake flour - *all-purpose flour*
2 tsp baking powder
½ tsp salt

Lemon icing glaze
320g (2 cups) powdered sugar
2 tbsp lemon juice
1 tsp salted butter - *melted*

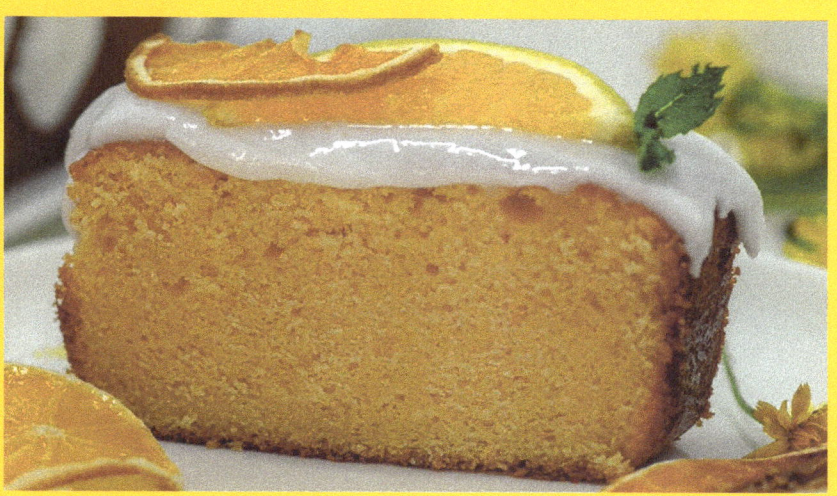

Method

1. Preheat oven to 170 °C fan forced. Grease a standard loaf cake pan and set aside.
2. In a large mixing bowl, beat together butter and sugar until creamy and smooth. Beat in eggs, one at a time until fully combined. Mix in the orange zest and juice until combined.
3. In a separate bowl, whisk together the flour, baking powder and salt. Add into the butter mixture and stir until mixed in well.
4. Spoon into prepared loaf cake pan, smoothing out the top. Bake for 55 minutes, or until a skewer inserted into the middle comes out clean. Remove from the oven and let it cool completely. Turn out onto a rack.

Making the glaze
5. In a large mixing bowl, combine sugar, lemon juice. Whisk until no lumps. Add the butter then whisk together until smooth.
6. Coat the orange loaf cake with icing glaze when fully cooled.

Recipe notes
7. You can adjust the consistency of the glaze to your liking by adding more powdered sugar or juice, to thicken or thin out.

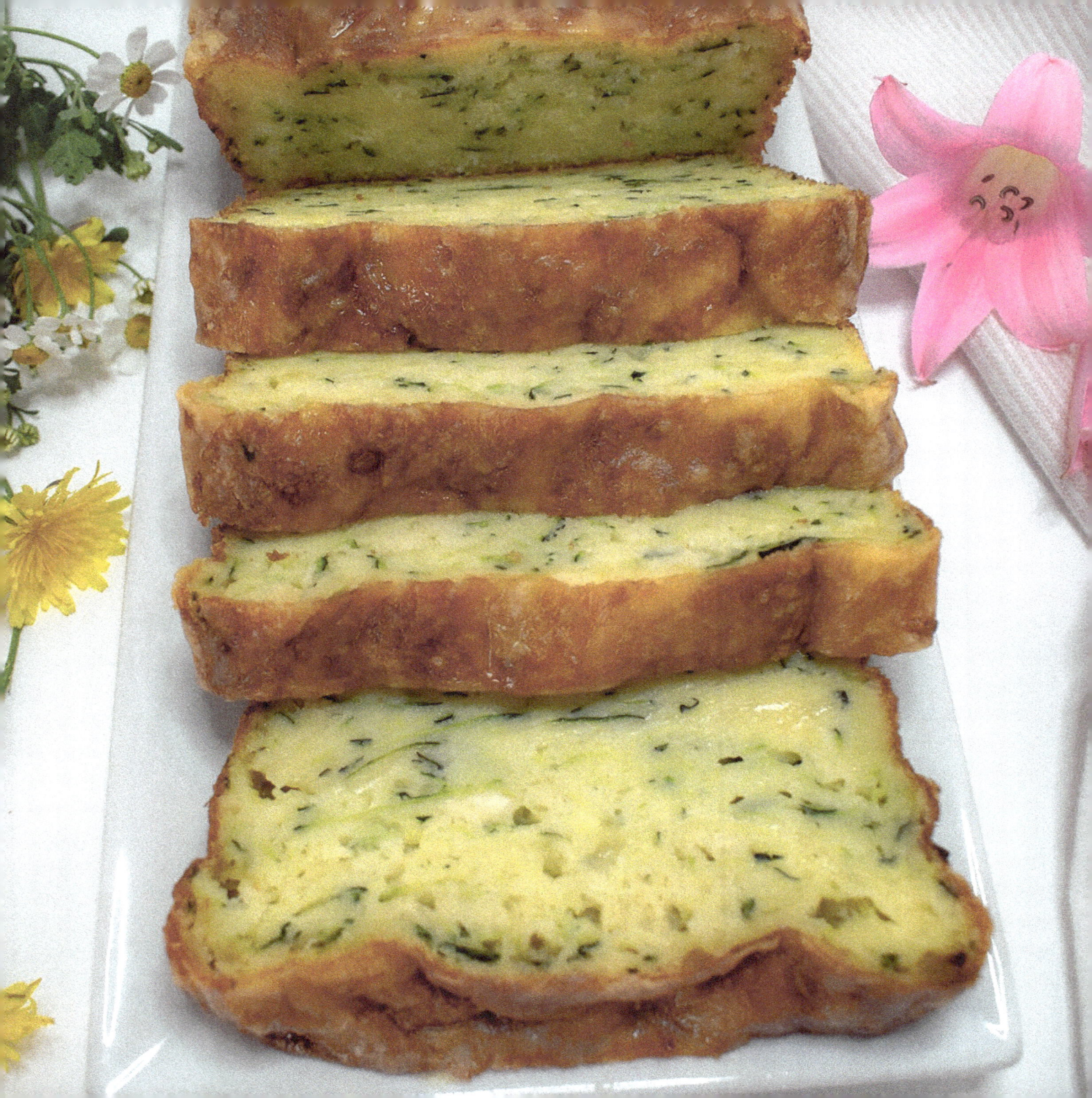

ZUCCHINI CHEESE BREAD – NO YEAST

A simple zucchini bread that's bursting with delicious cheese

Ingredients

Zucchini and Cheese
3 medium zucchinis - *400g grated*
1 ½ tsp salt
250g /10 slices Swiss cheese – *or similar such as mozzarella*

Dry ingredients
413g (2¾ cups) all-purpose flour
2 tsp baking powder
½ tsp baking soda
½ tsp salt

Wet Ingredients
375ml (1¼ cups) milk
28g (⅛ cup) butter - *melted*
2 tbsp vegetable oil
3 eggs - *at room temperature*
3 cloves garlic - *crushed*
1 tbsp white wine vinegar

Method

1. Grate the zucchini with box grater, measure about 400g (approx. 2½ cups), place in the bowl, sprinkle with salt and leave for 20 minutes.
2. Squeeze handfuls to remove the excess water, and place zucchini in mixing bowl, set aside.
3. Preheat oven to 170 °C fan forced. Grease a loaf pan with butter.
4. Place the dry ingredient in a mixing bowl. Whisk until combined.
5. Place the wet ingredients in another mixing bowl. Whisk until combined.
6. Make a well centre of the dry ingredients. Pour in the wet mixture until flour is incorporated and quickly stir through the zucchini.
7. Spread 1/3 of the batter in the loaf pan. Top with 5 slices of cheese.
8. Spread over another 1/3 of the batter, top with 5 slices of cheese, then finish with the remaining batter. Smooth top.
9. Bake for 50 minutes or until skewer inserted into the centre comes out clean. Brush with melted butter.
10. Allow the pan to cool for 10 minutes then transfer to a rack to cool another 30 minutes before slicing.

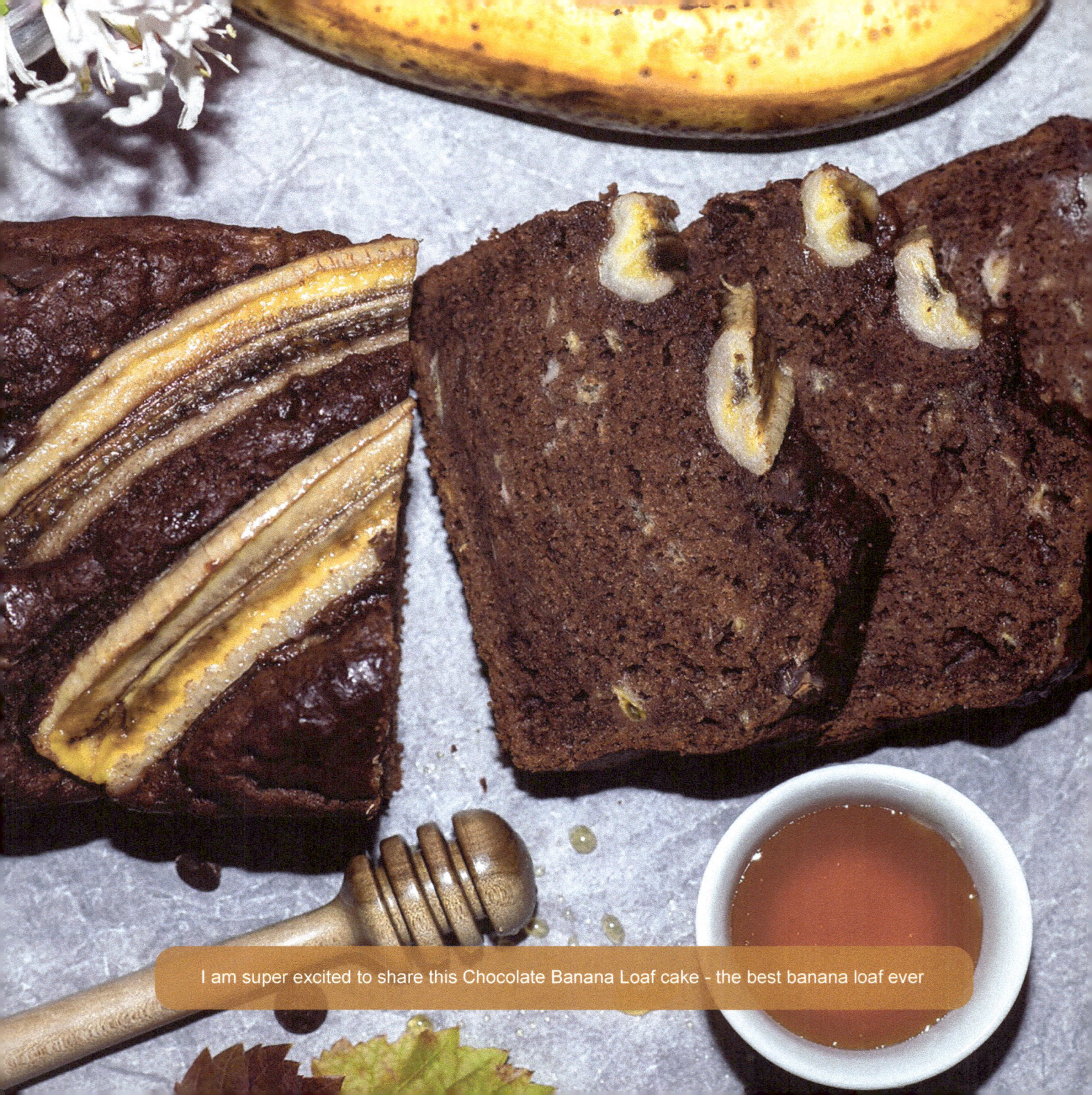

I am super excited to share this Chocolate Banana Loaf cake - the best banana loaf ever

MOIST BANANA CHOCOLATE LOAF

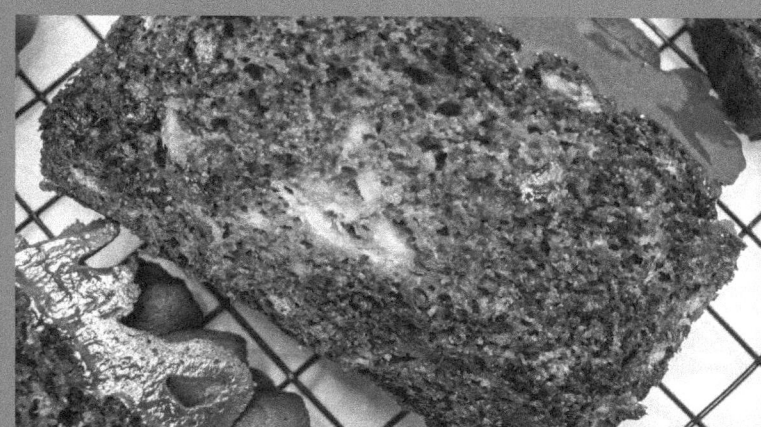

Ingredients

150g (1 cup) all-purpose flour
50g (½ cup) Dutch process cocoa
1 tsp baking soda
½ tsp salt
¼ tsp vegetable oil
3 large ripe bananas – *2 for mashing and one whole for the topping*
56g (¼ cup) unsalted butter
165g (¾ cup) brown sugar
2 large eggs - *at room temperature*
1 tsp pure vanilla extract
85g chocolate chips – *semi-sweet*

Method

1. Preheat oven to 170 °C fan forced. Grease a 9" by 5" loaf pan with nonstick cooking spray and set aside.

2. In a medium bowl, whisk together the flour, cocoa powder, baking soda and salt.

3. In a large bowl, mash the ripe bananas with a fork. Add the melted butter and oil and stir until combined. Stir into the brown sugar, egg, vanilla extract and mix until smooth.

4. Stir the dry ingredients into the wet ingredients, don't overmix. Stir in the semi-sweet chocolate chips.

5. Pour the batter into prepared pan. Bake for 50 minutes, or until a skewer inserted into the centre of the bread comes out with a few moist crumbs.

6. Remove the pan from the oven and set on a wire cooling rack. Let the bread cool in the pan for 15 minutes. Run a knife around the edges of the bread and carefully remove from the pan.

7. Cut into slices and serve.

Note: Feel free to enrich the flavour with a topping of chocolate ganache if desired (see page 109)".

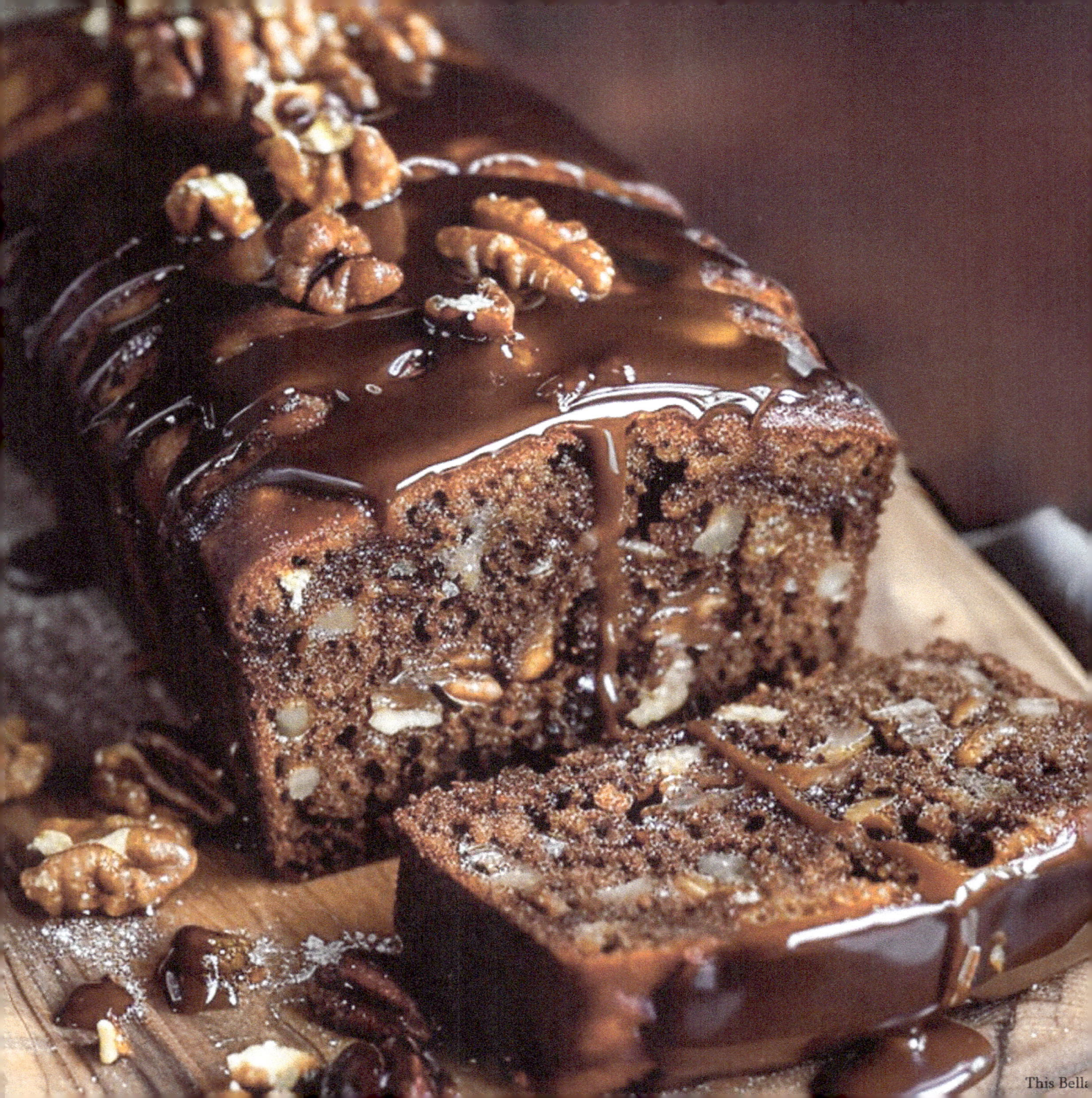

ESPRESSO AND DATE LOAF

Ingredients

The loaf

263g (1¾) cups flour
1 tsp baking soda
½ tsp baking powder
¼ tsp salt
½ tsp ground cinnamon
¼ tsp ground nutmeg
220g (1 cup) sugar
113g (½ cup) unsalted butter - *softened*
3 eggs
1 tsp vanilla extract
1 cup chopped pecans
233g (1½ cups) dates - *pitted and chopped*
1 cup hot espresso

The espresso glaze

160g (1 cup) powdered sugar
2 tbsp espresso
1 tsp vanilla extract

Method

1. Preheat oven to 170°C fan forced. Grease and flour a 9 x 5 inch loaf tin.
2. In a bowl combine chopped dates and hot espresso. Let it sit for 15 minutes to soften the dates
3. In another bowl sift all dry ingredients, flour, baking soda, baking powder, salt, cinnamon, nutmeg
4. In a large bowl beat butter and sugar until light and fluffy and add eggs, one at the time. Beat until well combined and stir in vanilla extract
5. Gradually add the flour mixture to the batter mixture just until combined. Stir in softened dates with remaining liquid and add the chopped pecans
6. Pour the batter into the prepared loaf tin and smooth the top
7. Bake for 60 minutes or until the skewer inserted to the centre comes out clean
8. Allow the loaf to cool in the tin for 10 minutes then transfer to a wire rack to cool completely.

Glaze

9. In a small bowl, whisk together powdered sugar, espresso and vanilla extract until smooth. Drizzle the espresso glaze over the cooked loaf. Let it sit in fridge for 30 minutes before slicing and serving.

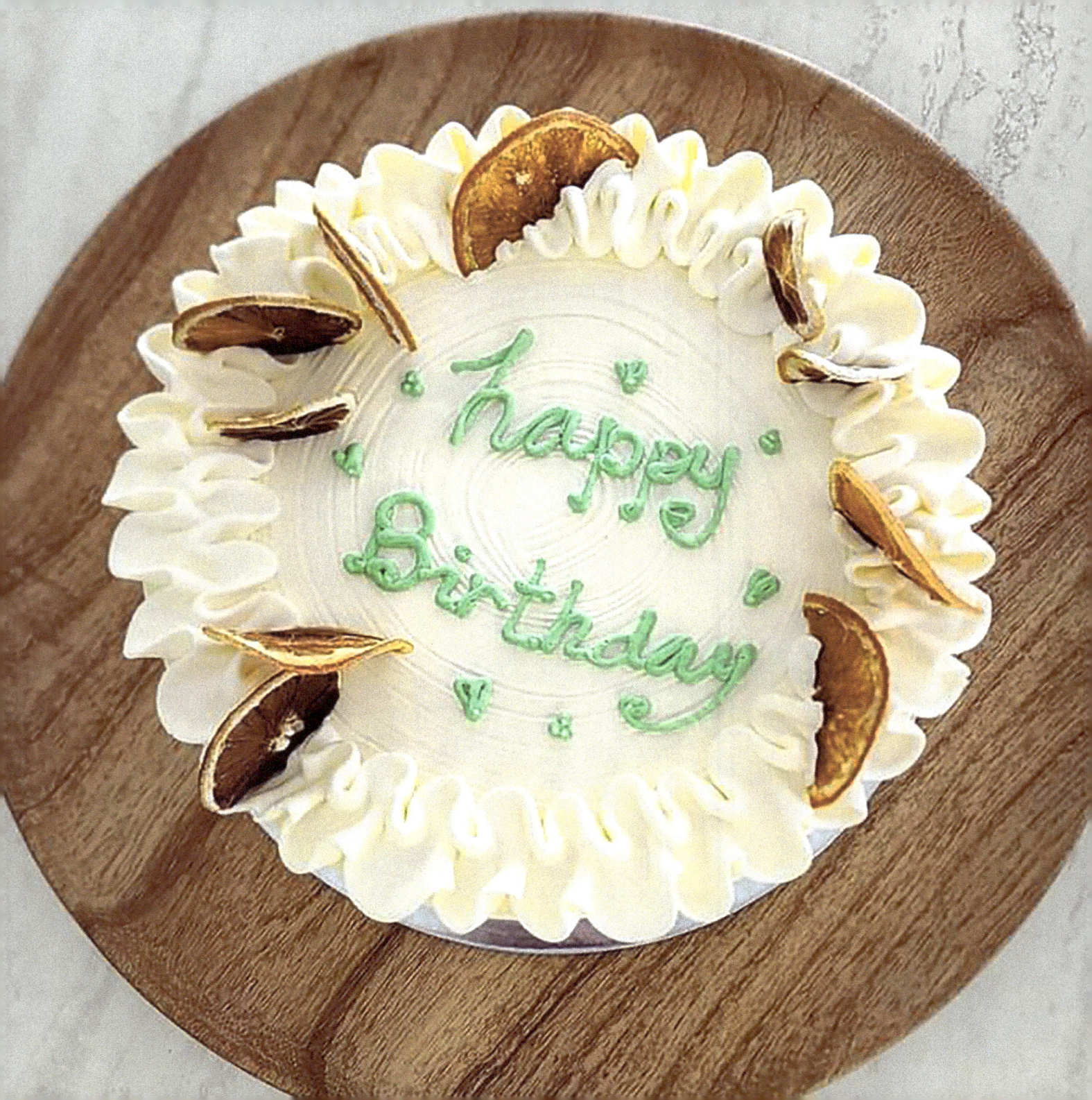

LEMON CAKE

Ingredients

225g (1½ cups) self-raising flour

½ tsp salt

170g (¾ cup butter) - *softened*

220g (1 cup) raw caster sugar

1 tbsp lemon zest

3 eggs - *room temperature*

60ml (4 tbsp) lemon juice

125ml (½ cup) milk

Method

1. Preheat oven to 180°C fan forced. Grease and line the base of an 8" baking tin with baking paper

2. Beat butter, lemon zest and sugar in a bowl until light and fluffy. Add eggs one at a time. The mixture will be light and creamy

3. Sift self-raising flour over the egg mixture, then add the lemon juice and beat for a few seconds. Continue while adding milk and beat until well combined

4. Pour in the prepared tin. Tap the tin on the worktop to settle the batter.

5. Bake in preheated oven approximately 50 minutes or until the skewer comes up clean.

6. Remove the cake from the oven and allow to cool. Dust with icing sugar

7. You can also decorate with lemon butter cream (see page 115) and fill with lemon curd (see page 108) as desired.

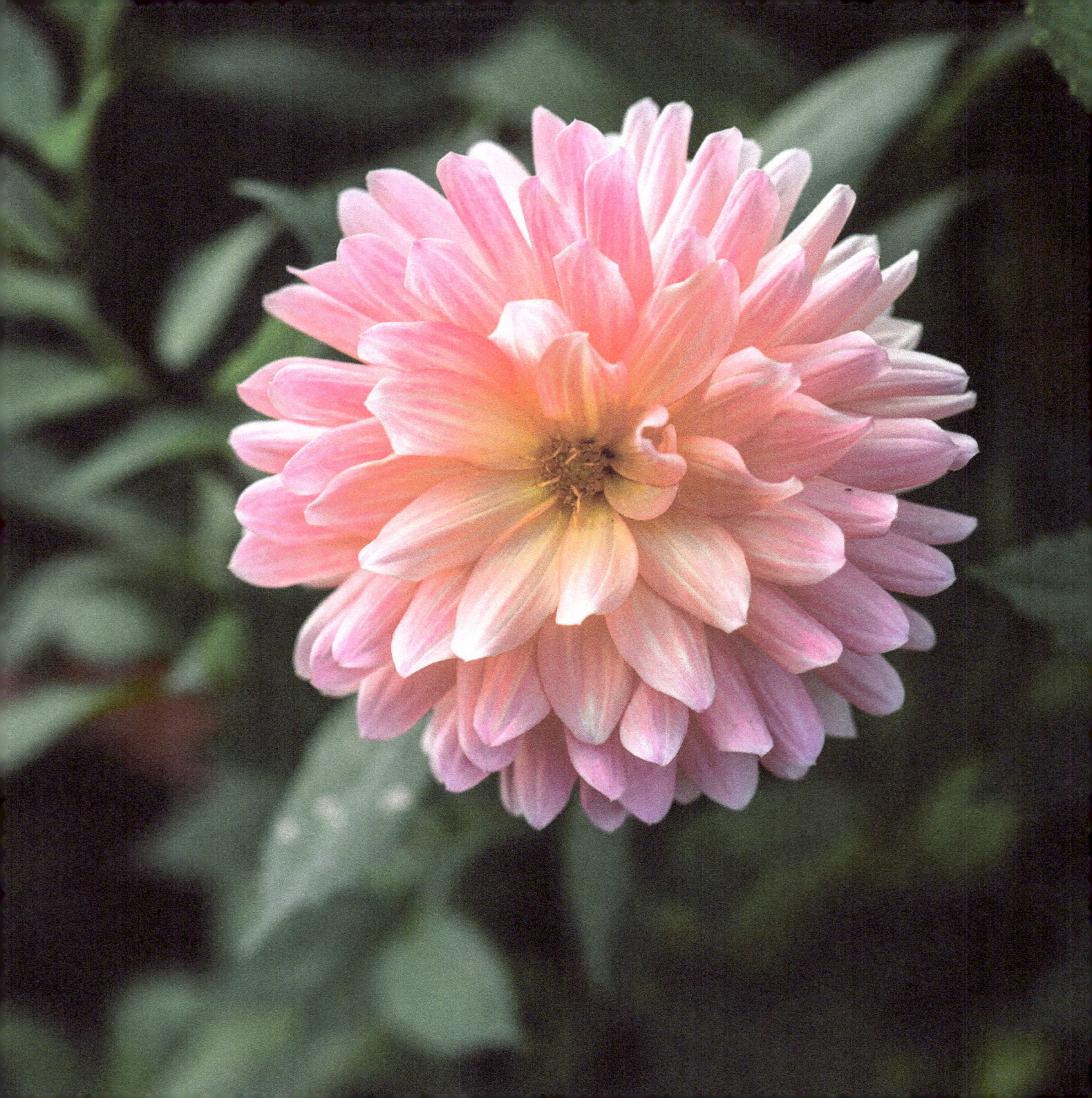

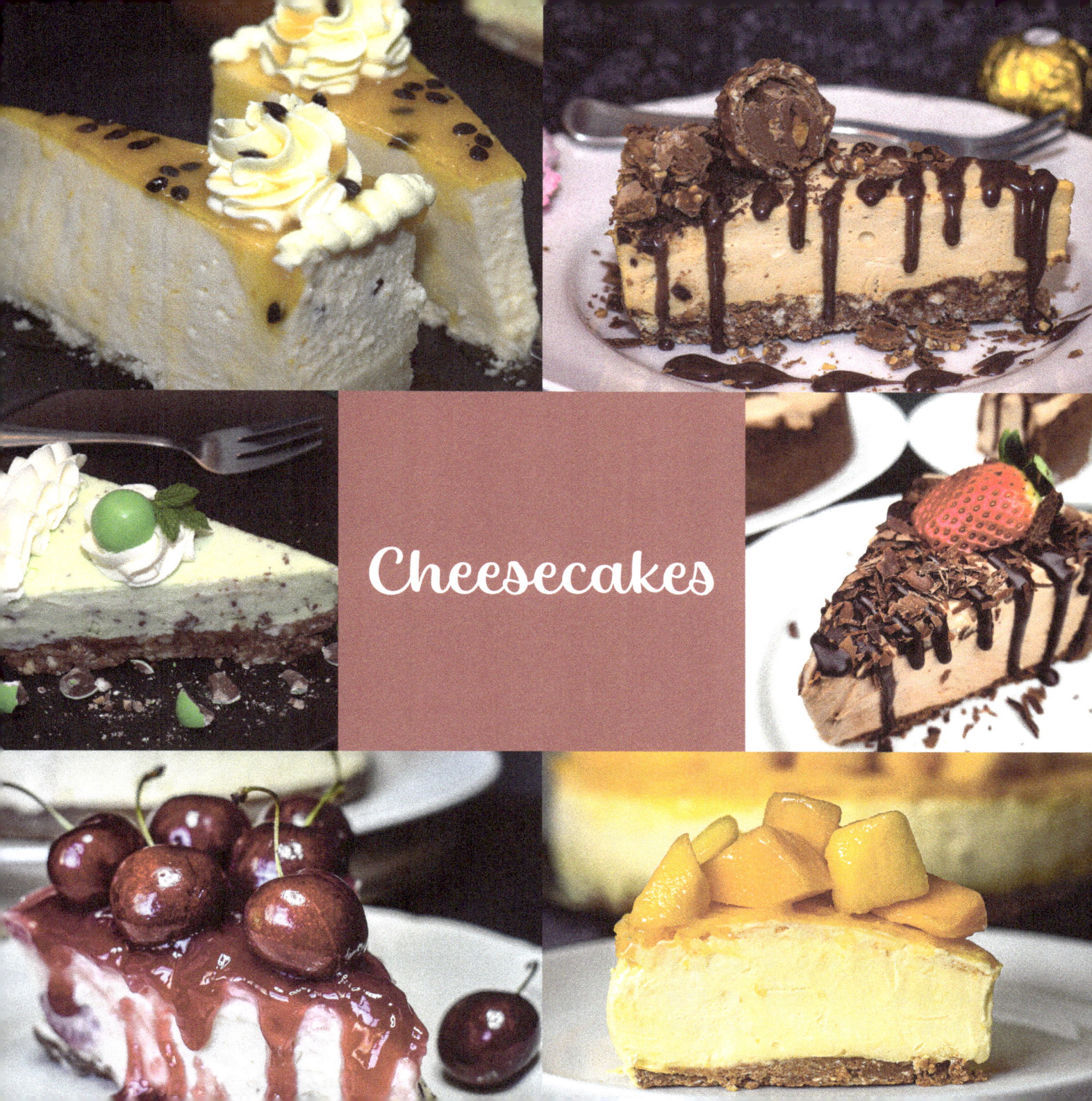

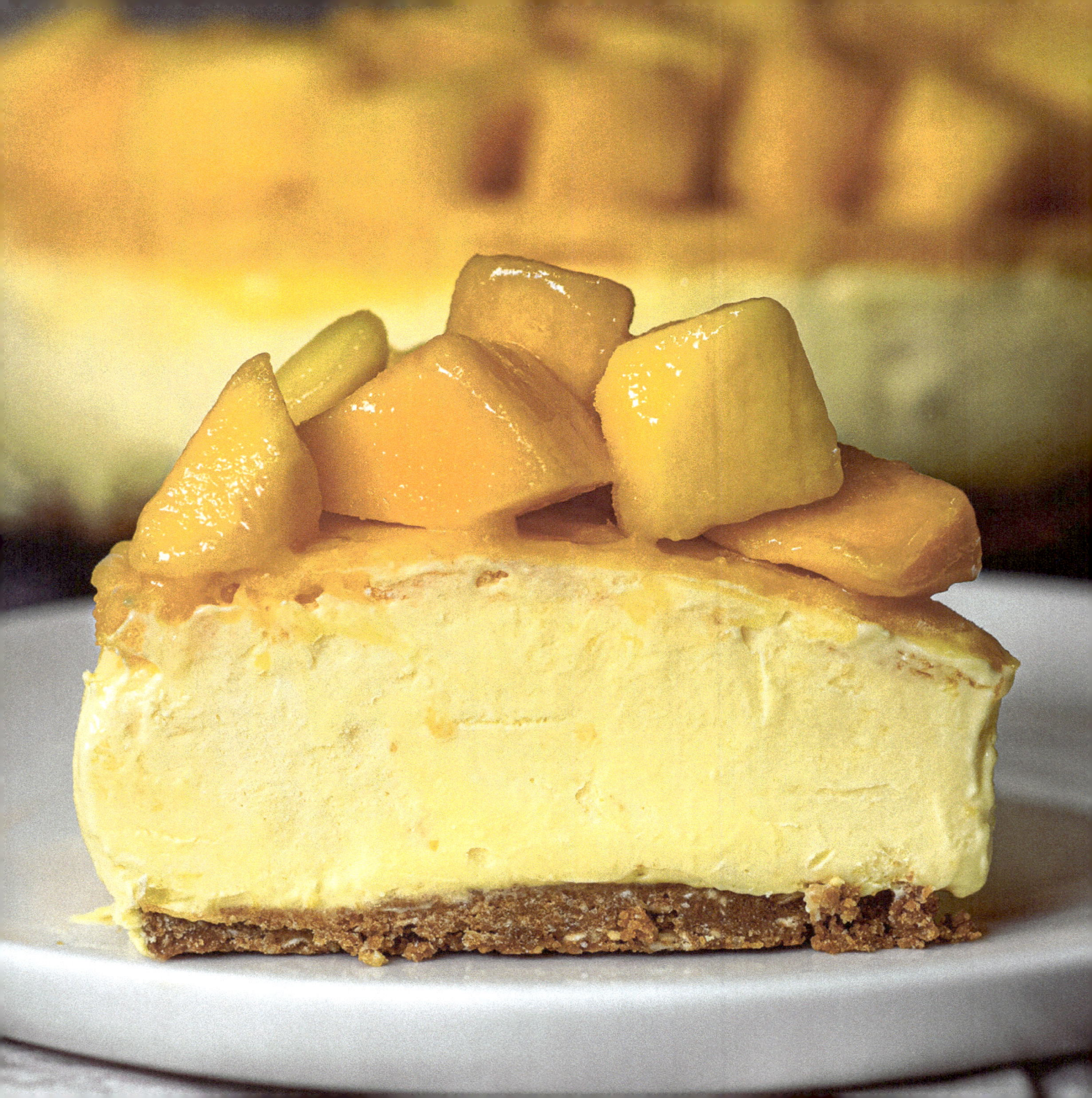

NO BAKE MANGO CHEESECAKE

Ingredients

Crust
180g (1½ cups) cracker crumbs
(Biscoff or similar)
55g (¼ cup) granulated sugar
113g (½ cup) unsalted butter - *melted*

Cheesecake filling
500g cream cheese (Philadelphia) - *softened*
1 tsp vanilla extract
160g (1 cup) powdered sugar
260g (1 cup) mango puree - *from fresh mangoes will taste better*
250ml (1 cup) thickened cream - *chilled*

Topping
Sliced mangoes

Method

Preparing the crust
1. In a mixing bowl, combine cracker crumbs, granulated sugar, and melted butter until the mixture resembles wet sand.
2. Press the mixture firmly into the 8-inch springform pan, forming an even layer.
3. Place the pan in refrigerator to chill while preparing the filling.

Making the cheesecake filling
4. In a large mixing bowl, beat the softened cream cheese until smooth and creamy.
5. Add powdered sugar and vanilla extract and beat until well combined.
6. Fold in the mango puree until evenly incorporated.
7. In a separate mixing bowl, whip the chilled heavy cream until stiff peaks form.
8. Combine filling and cream by gently folding the whipped cream into the mango cheesecake mixture until no streaks remain.

Assembly
9. Pour the mango cheesecake filling over the prepared crust in the springform pan, spreading it out evenly with a spatula.
10. Cover the cheesecake with plastic wrapping and refrigerate for at least 4 hours, or until set.

Garnish and serve
11. Before serving, garnish the top of the cheesecake with sliced mango if desired.
12. Run a knife around the edges of the cheesecake to loosen it from the pan, then release the springform sides.
13. Slice and serve the chill mango cheesecake, enjoying its creamy texture and refreshing mango flavour.

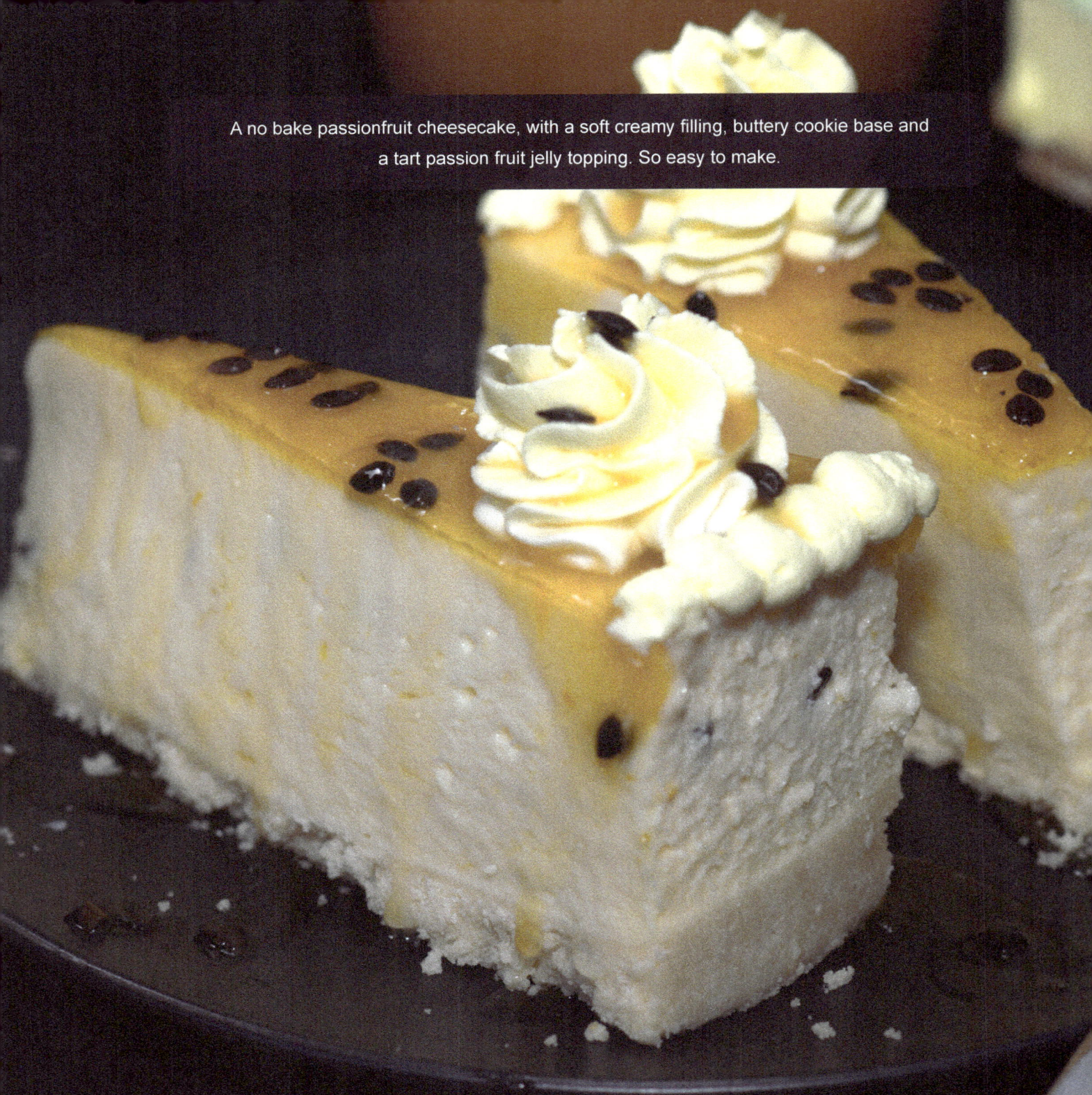
A no bake passionfruit cheesecake, with a soft creamy filling, buttery cookie base and a tart passion fruit jelly topping. So easy to make.

NO BAKE PASSION FRUIT CHEESECAKE

Ingredients

Crust
200g (1¾ cup) biscuits - *Arnott's or digestive biscuits*
74g (⅓ cup) unsalted butter - *melted*

Cheesecake filling
2 tsp powdered gelatine
250ml (1 cup) thickened cream
500g cream cheese - *softened*
125ml passion fruit pulp
124g (½ cup + 1 tbsp) caster sugar - *or condensed milk*

Passion fruit jelly
125ml (½ cup) water
1 tsp powdered gelatine
55g (¼ cup) caster sugar
125ml (½ cup) passionfruit pulp

Method

Preparing the crust
1. Grease the base and sides of an 8-inch springform pan and line with baking paper.
2. Blitz the biscuits in a blender to crumbs. Add melted butter and mix well.
3. Pour the mixture into the pan, using a glass to press it down firmly and evenly.

Making the cheesecake filling
4. Mix 2 teaspoons powdered gelatine in 1½ tablespoons boiling water until lump free. In a medium bowl, beat cream with a handheld electric beater or whisk to soft peaks. Place in the fridge.
5. In a large bowl beat the cream cheese and sugar with an electric beater, until smooth and lump free. Scrape down the sides. Add passionfruit pulp and gelatine mixture - beat until well combined. Lastly, gently fold in the cream, one third at a time.

Assembly
6. Pour the cheesecake filling over the prepared crust, spreading it out evenly with a spatula. Be sure to push it up against all the sides. This will stop the jelly from seeping down the sides when added. Chill, while you make the topping.

Making the passionfruit jelly
7. In a small saucepan add water and sprinkle over the gelatine. Let it soften for 2 minutes, then place over a low heat, stirring constantly until gelatine has dissolved. Add sugar and continue stirring until a clear syrup. Remove from heat and stir in passionfruit pulp. Allow the jelly to cool for 10 minutes.
8. Pour the passionfruit jelly over the cheesecake and return it to fridge to chill for at least 6 hours

Removing the Cheesecake and serving
9. Use a knife to gently ease the paper from the sides of the pan. Release and remove the outer ring. Peel away the paper from the edges. Using the paper under the cheesecake, gently lift it up off the pan base. Slide a large spatula between the paper and cheesecake to release it completely. Slide the cheesecake off the paper and onto a serving plate. Slice and serve.

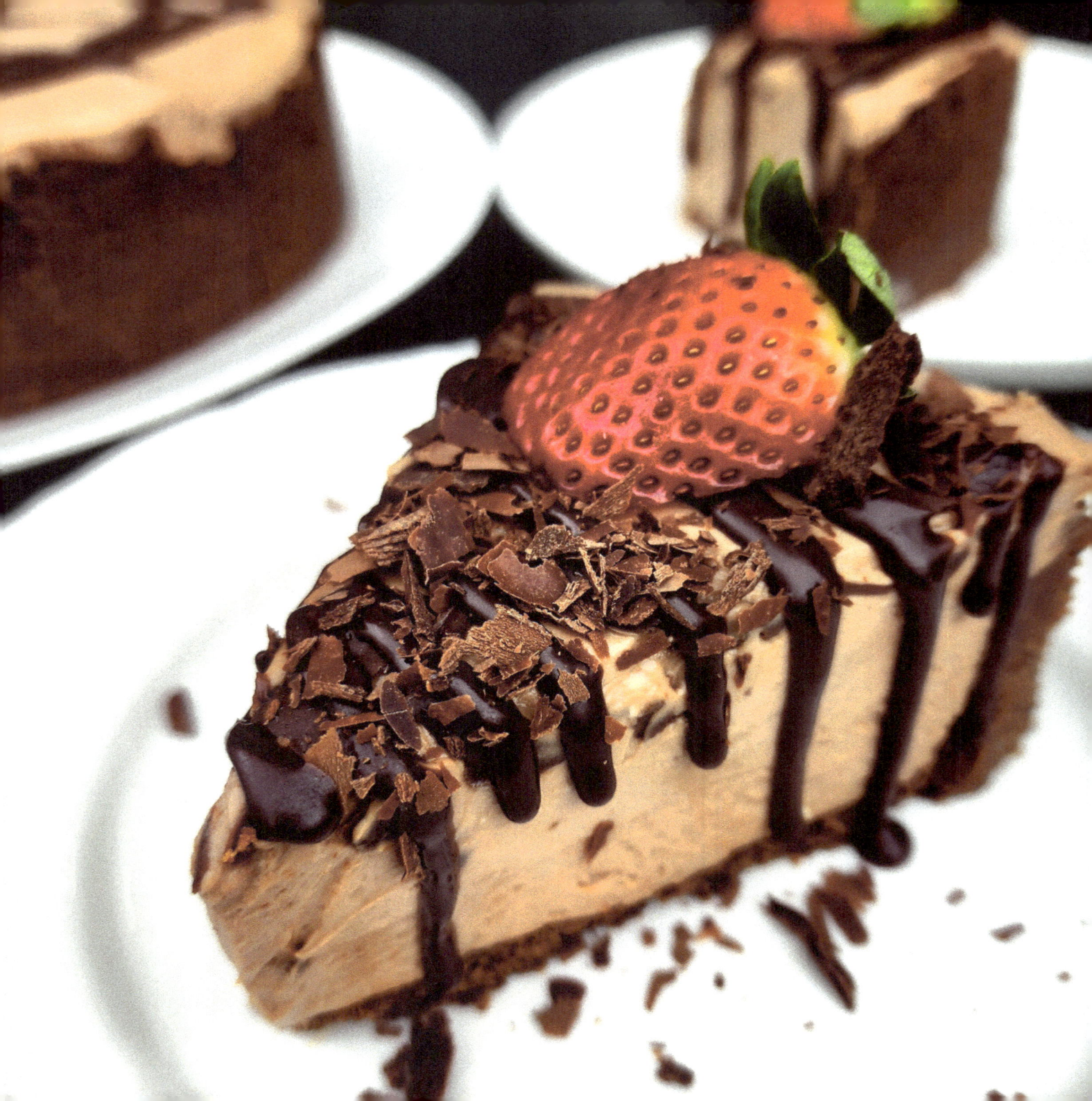

NO BAKE BAILEY'S CHOCOLATE CHEESECAKE

Ingredients

Base

250g chocolate ripple biscuits
113g (½ cup) butter - *melted*

Filling

500g cream cheese – *Philadelphia recommended*
160g (1 cup) icing sugar
60ml espresso
100ml (½ cup) chocolate ganache
313ml (1¼ cups) thickened cream
1 tsp vanilla extract
4 tbsp Baileys' Irish Cream

Topping

Chocolate ganache – *please see page 109*
Chocolate shard – *please see page 110*

Method

Preparing the base

1. Prepare an 8-inch springform pan by lightly greasing the edges and the bottom of the pan with cooking spray. Line with parchment paper.
2. Grind the biscuits into fine crumbs using a food processor or blender. Pour the melted butter over the biscuit crumbs and stir until crumbs are well coated
3. Pour the crumb mix into the springform pan and press firmly into the bottom and the sides to create a thick crust. Refrigerate the crust while preparing the filling.

Preparing the filling

4. In a microwave safe bowl, combine the chocolate and ¼ cup of heavy thickened cream until the chocolate has melted, stirring occasionally
5. Beat the cream cheese until its completely smooth, scrape down the sides of the bowl as needed. Add sugar, vanilla, espresso and Baileys - beating until smooth. Then add the melted chocolate and thickened cream, beating until it's completely combined
6. Pour the filling into prepared crust, spreading evenly. Refrigerate for 4 hours minimum or overnight for better results.
7. Remove from the pan and decorate as desired.

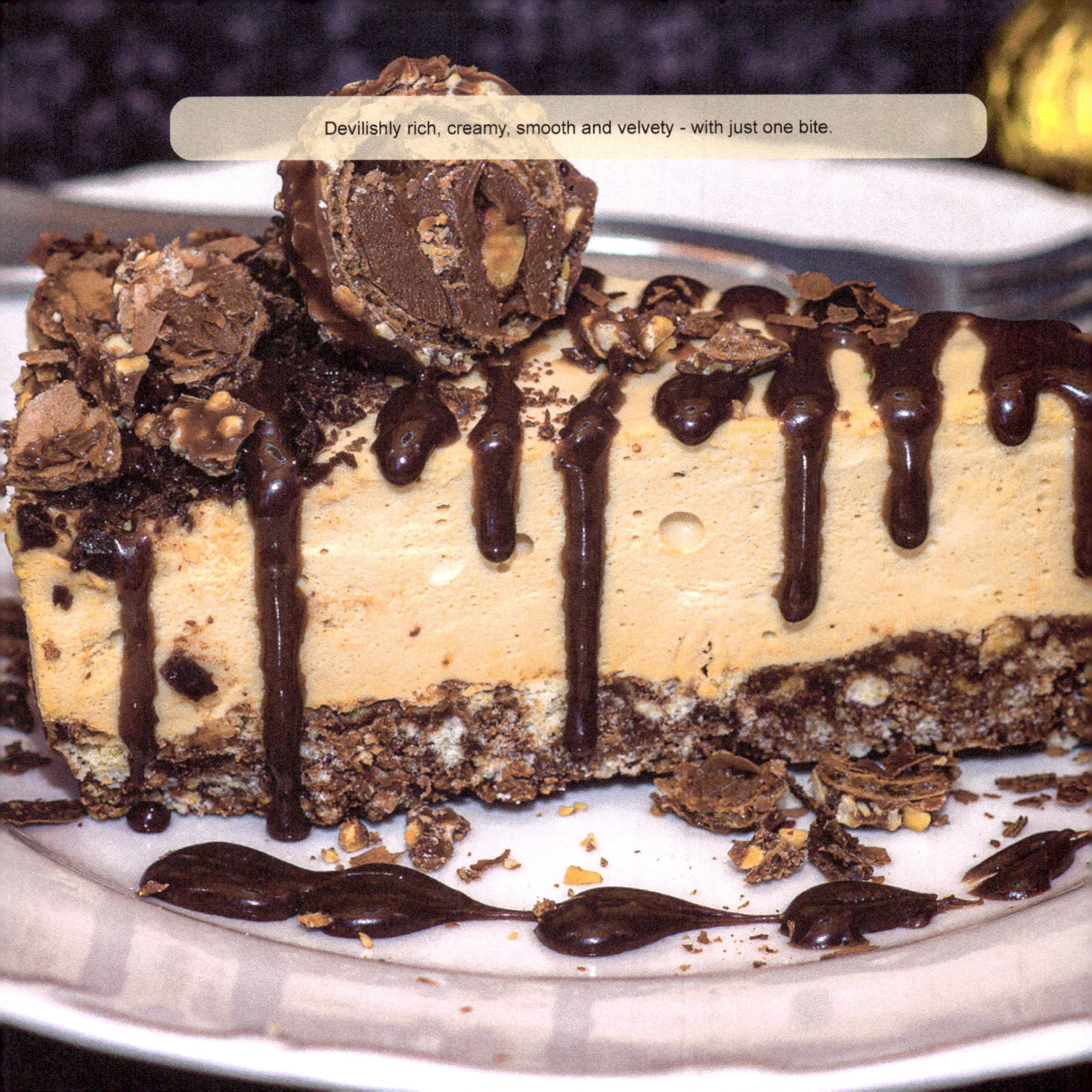

Devilishly rich, creamy, smooth and velvety - with just one bite.

FERRERO ROCHER COFFEE CHEESECAKE

Ingredients

The base
290g (1½ cups) Gaham Crackers crumbs
30g (1 cup) Rice Krispies cereal - *slightly crushed*
75g (½ cup) roasted hazelnuts - *finely chopped*
19g (3 tbsp) cocoa powder
55g (¼ cup) granulated sugar
113g (½ cup) butter - *at room temperature*

Coffee filling
2 x 250g packages cream cheese - *full fat*
250ml (1 cup) sour cream
165g (¾ cup) granulated sugar
83ml (⅓ cup) thickened cream
1 tbsp vanilla extract
4 large eggs - *room temperature*
3 tbsp corn starch
2 tsp coffee flavour espresso

Garnish
Ferrero Rocher chocolates

Method

Making the crust
1. Line the bottom of an 8" springform pan with parchment paper. Mix Graham cracker crumbs, rice Krispies, cocoa powder, chopped hazelnuts and sugar in a large mixing bowl.
2. Melt butter in a separate bowl and add to ingredients. Mix until combined. Press the mixture firmly into the pan, forming an even layer.

Making the cheese filling
3. Preheat oven to 160° fan forced. Boil 4 cups of water – to use later for a bain-marie (water bath)
4. Mix cream cheese, sour cream, granulated sugar, thicken cream and vanilla extract in a food processor or Thermomix until a smooth, creamy texture - completely lump free.
5. Add eggs and continue processing. Scrape the sides well, add corn starch and continue mixing. Finally add coffee extract, mixing until all is thoroughly combined.

Assembly
6. Place the pan on a sheet of aluminium foil and fold the foil over so the pan is completely covered to prevent water from getting into the pan. Place into a bain-marie (large dish)
7. Pour the cheesecake mix into the pan, spreading it evenly over the crust.
8. Carefully pour boiling water into the bain-marie filling it to about ¾ full.
9. Place into the middle rack of the oven. Bake for 25 minutes at 160°C, then decrease to 120°C and bake another 75 minutes.
10. Turn the oven off and crack the door open about an inch. Leave the cake in the oven for about 1 hour - so it's cool enough to touch, then carefully slide it out.
11. When it's cooled completely, run a thin spatula or knife around the rim. Refrigerate, uncovered for at least 6 hours. Carefully remove the outer ring leaving the cheesecake on the parchment paper.

Garnish and serve
12. If desired, you can add a dripping of ganache and Ferrero Rocher as toppers.

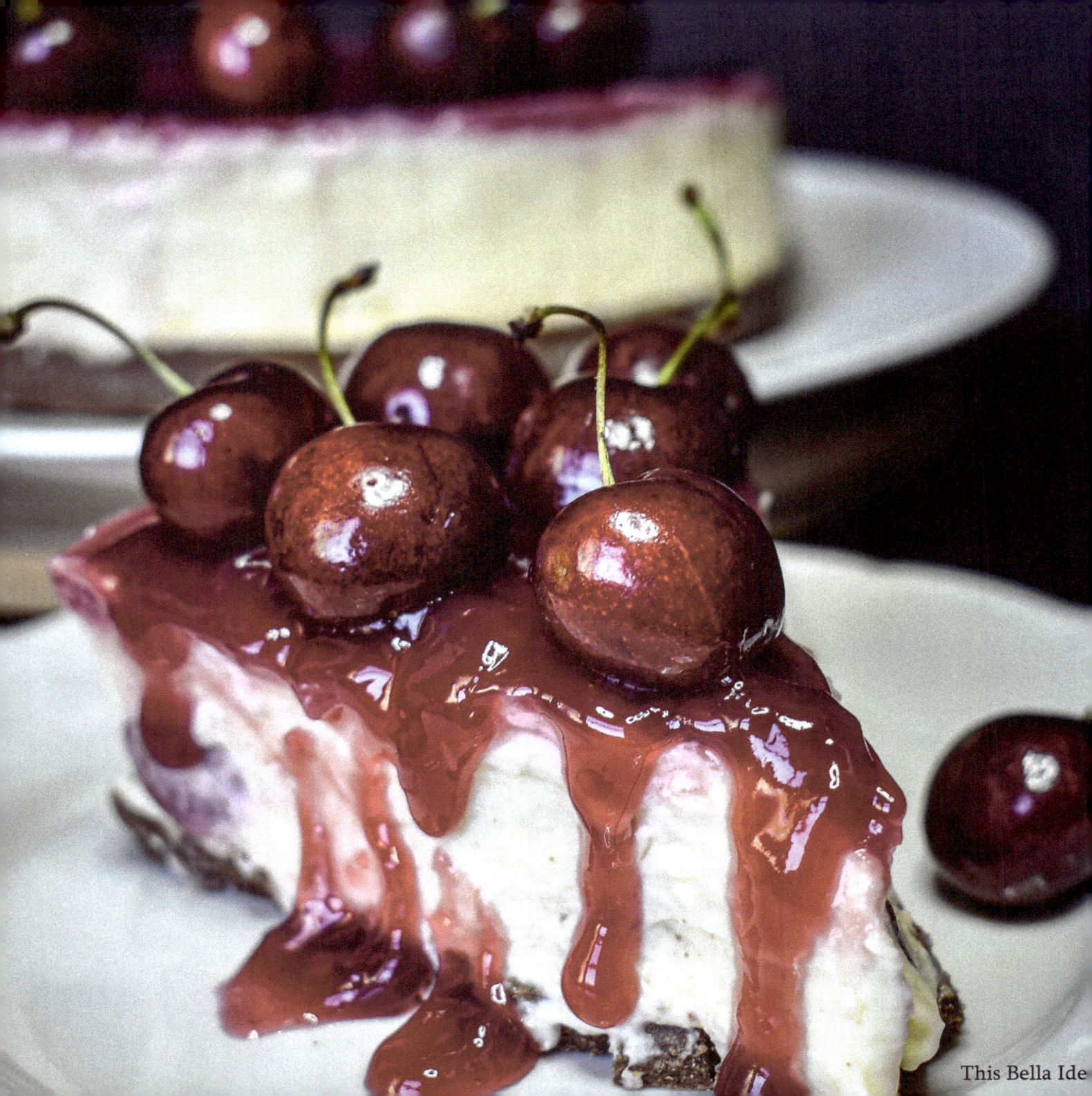

NO BAKE BLACKFOREST CHEESECAKE

Rich, velvety, delicious and easy to prepare. This no bake black forest cheesecake is the absolutely perfect dessert.

Ingredients

Crust

250g chocolate biscuits
100g (0.4 cup) butter - *melted*

Cheesecake filling

2 tsp gelatine
63ml (0.4 cup) water
500g cream cheese (I use Philadelphia) - *softened*
145g (⅔ cup) caster sugar
1 tbsp lemon juice
313g (1¼ cups) thickened cream
425g pitted morello cherries

The topping

1 tbsp corn flour
1 tbsp caster sugar
2 tbsp red wine

Method

Preparing the crust

1. Using a food processor, process biscuits until the mixture is finely crumbed, add melted butter, process until well combined. Press biscuits mixture evenly over the base and sides of a 20 cm spring form pan, refrigerate for about 20 minutes

Making the cheesecake filling

2. Sprinkle gelatine over the water in small heat proof container and put in microwave for 15 seconds. Stir until gelatine is dissolved and set at room temperature
3. Beat cream cheese, sugar and lemon juice in a small bowl with electric mixer until smooth
4. Whip thicken cream until soft peaks form, then fold into the cheese mixture in 3 batches, then continue folding in the gelatine mixture.
5. Drain the morello cherries over a bowl and reserve ¾ cup of the syrup. Dry the cherries on absorbent paper.

Assembly

6. Spoon ⅓ of the cheesecake mixture into crumbed crust, top with half of the morello cherries. Repeat the layering and ending with cheese mixture on top. Refrigerate until just firm
7. Meanwhile, make the topping: Combine the corn flour and sugar with the reserved cherry's syrup in a small saucepan. Stir over heat until mixture boils and thickens, stir in red wine, let it cool
8. Spread the topping over the topping cheesecake and refrigerate overnight.
9. Serve with fresh cherries and a dollop of whipped cream.

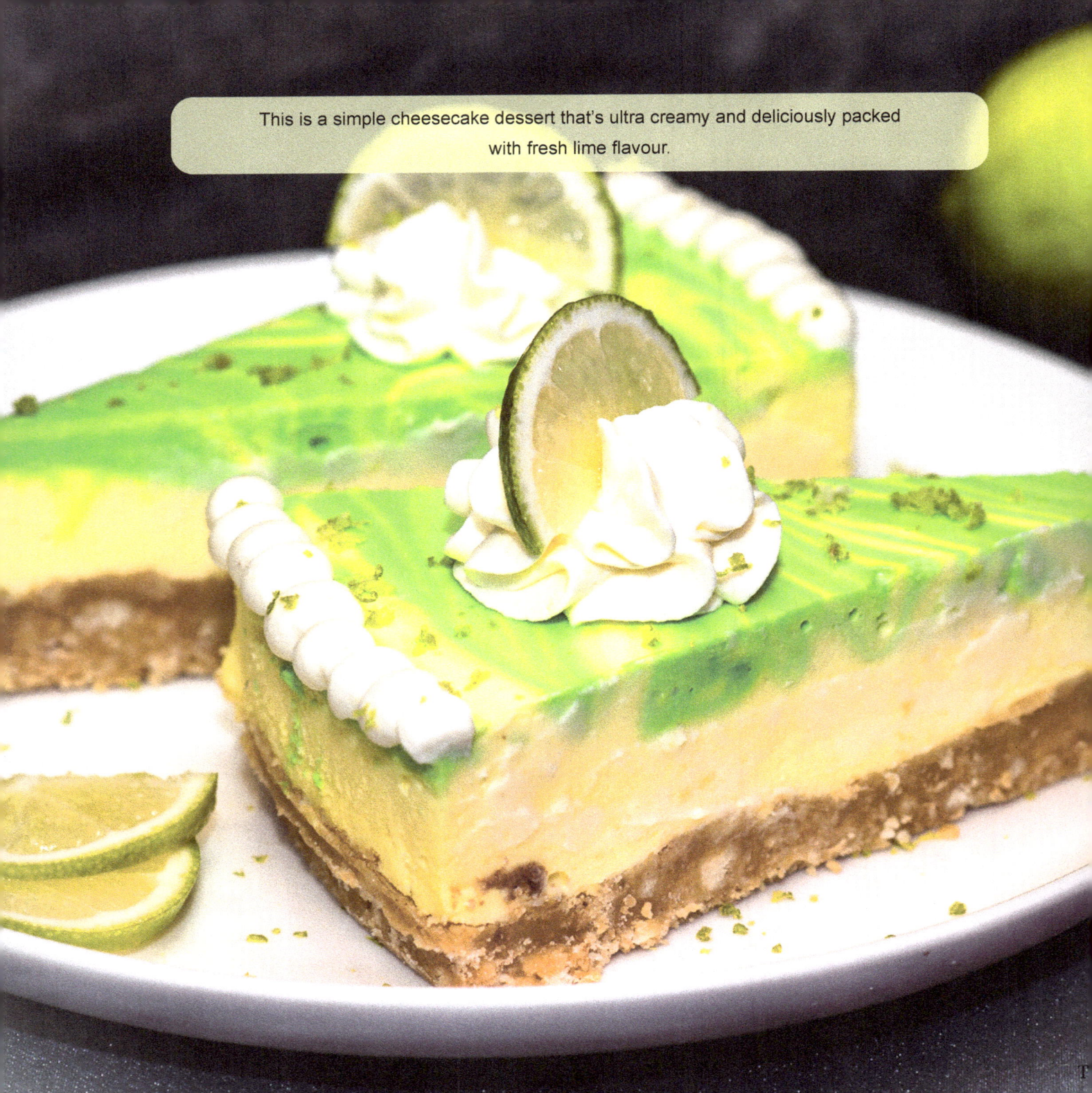

This is a simple cheesecake dessert that's ultra creamy and deliciously packed with fresh lime flavour.

NO BAKE LIME CHEESECAKE

Ingredients

160g (1½ cups) Graham crackers - *crumbed*

70g (5 tbsp) unsalted butter - *melted*

Cheesecake filling

500g cream cheese

200g (1¼ cups) powdered sugar

Juice and zest of 2 limes

313g (1¼ cups) thickened cream

1 tsp Vanilla extract

For decorating

Thickened cream and lime slices for garnish

Method

Making the crust

1. Combine the Graham crackers crumbs and melted butter until moist and crumbly
2. Press the mixture into the bottom of 9-inch spring form pan and refrigerate to set.

Making the cheesecake filling

3. Combine the cream cheese, powdered sugar and vanilla extract in a large bowl, mixing with hand mixer on medium speed, until smooth.
4. Add the lime juice and zest and mix well until incorporated.
5. Fold in the thickened cream and mix for about 3 minutes - until the mixture is fluffy and creamy and there are no streaks in the batter.

Assembly

6. Pour the cheesecake mixture into the prepared crust and smooth out the top with a spatula.
7. Refrigerate to set for 6 hours or overnight.

For serving

8. Pipe with whipped cream and add some lime slices and lime zest for garnish (optional).

Note: If you want to create a fancy lime cheesecake, add some green food colouring to the cheesecake mixture, using a knife to swirl the mixture together.

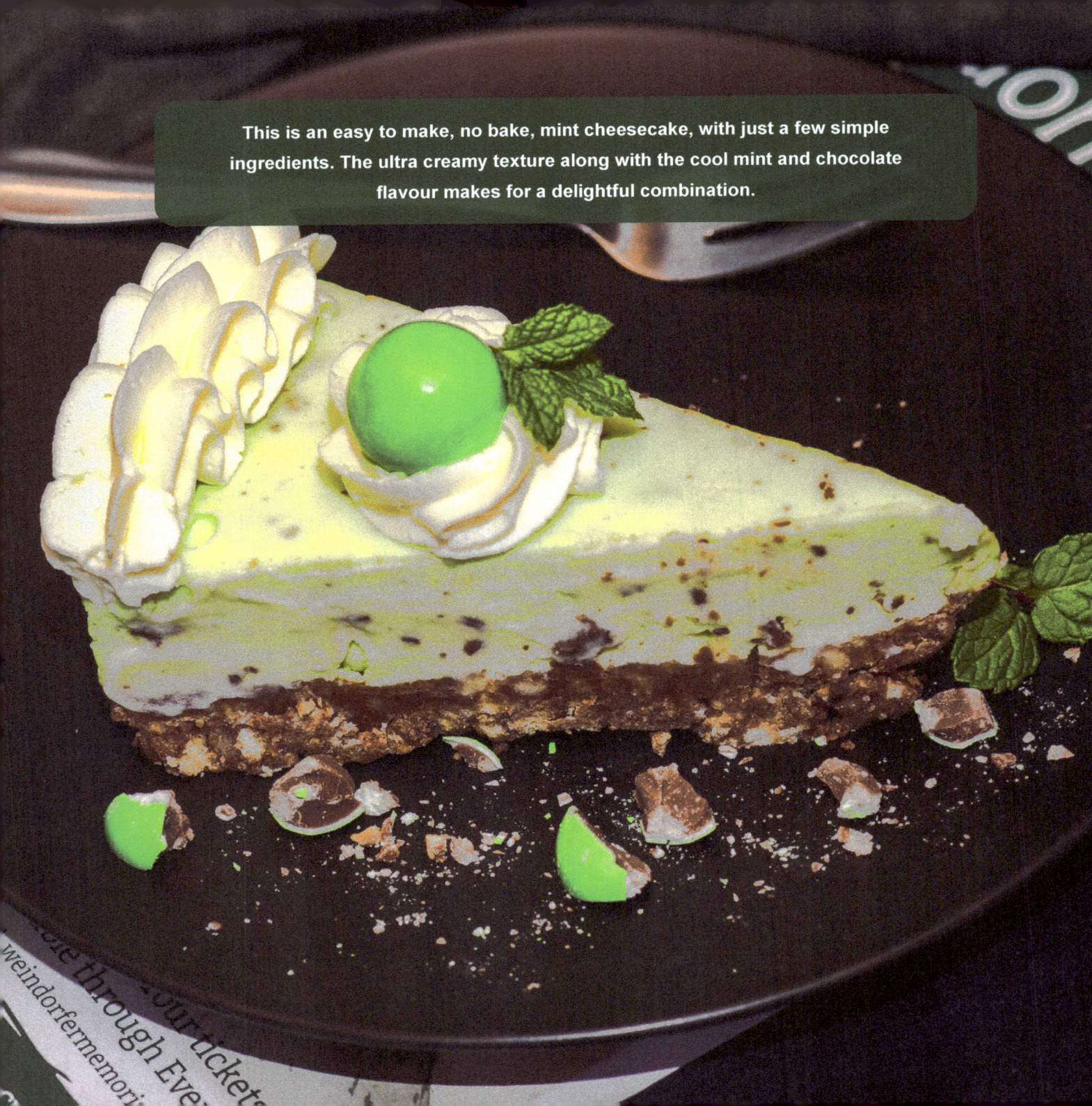

This is an easy to make, no bake, mint cheesecake, with just a few simple ingredients. The ultra creamy texture along with the cool mint and chocolate flavour makes for a delightful combination.

NO BAKE MINT CHEESECAKE

Ingredients

Crust

150g (1¼ cups) crushed Oreo cookies, or Biscoff biscuits

74g (⅓ cup) butter - *melted*

Cheesecake filling

500g cream cheese

160g (1 cup) powdered sugar

250ml (1 cup) thickened cream - *whipped until stiff*

A few drops peppermint extract

85g mini chocolate chips

Method

Preparing the crust

1. Grease the line base and sides of 8-inch springform pan with baking paper.
2. Add crushed Oreo cookies and the melted butter to a mixing bowl and mix with a fork until combined.
3. Press the Oreo cookie mixture into the bottom of a spring-form pan and up the sides of the pan about 2/3 of the height of the pan.
4. Set the crust aside to chill in the fridge while making the cheesecake filling.

Making the cheesecake filling

5. Add the cream cheese to a large bowl and whip until smooth, continue mixing while adding the powdered sugar.
6. Fold in whipped cream and green food colouring.
7. Add peppermint extract and mini chocolate chips and fold until just combined.

Assembly

8. Pour the cheesecake mixture over the chilled crust, pressing it evenly into the bottom and sides of the pan and smoothing it out on the top to prevent air bubbles.
9. Chill the cheesecake for 24 hours in the fridge before serving, alternatively chill in the freezer for 2 hours or overnight.

Serving

10. Serve with a dollop of whipped cream and crushed minty crunchy chocolate.

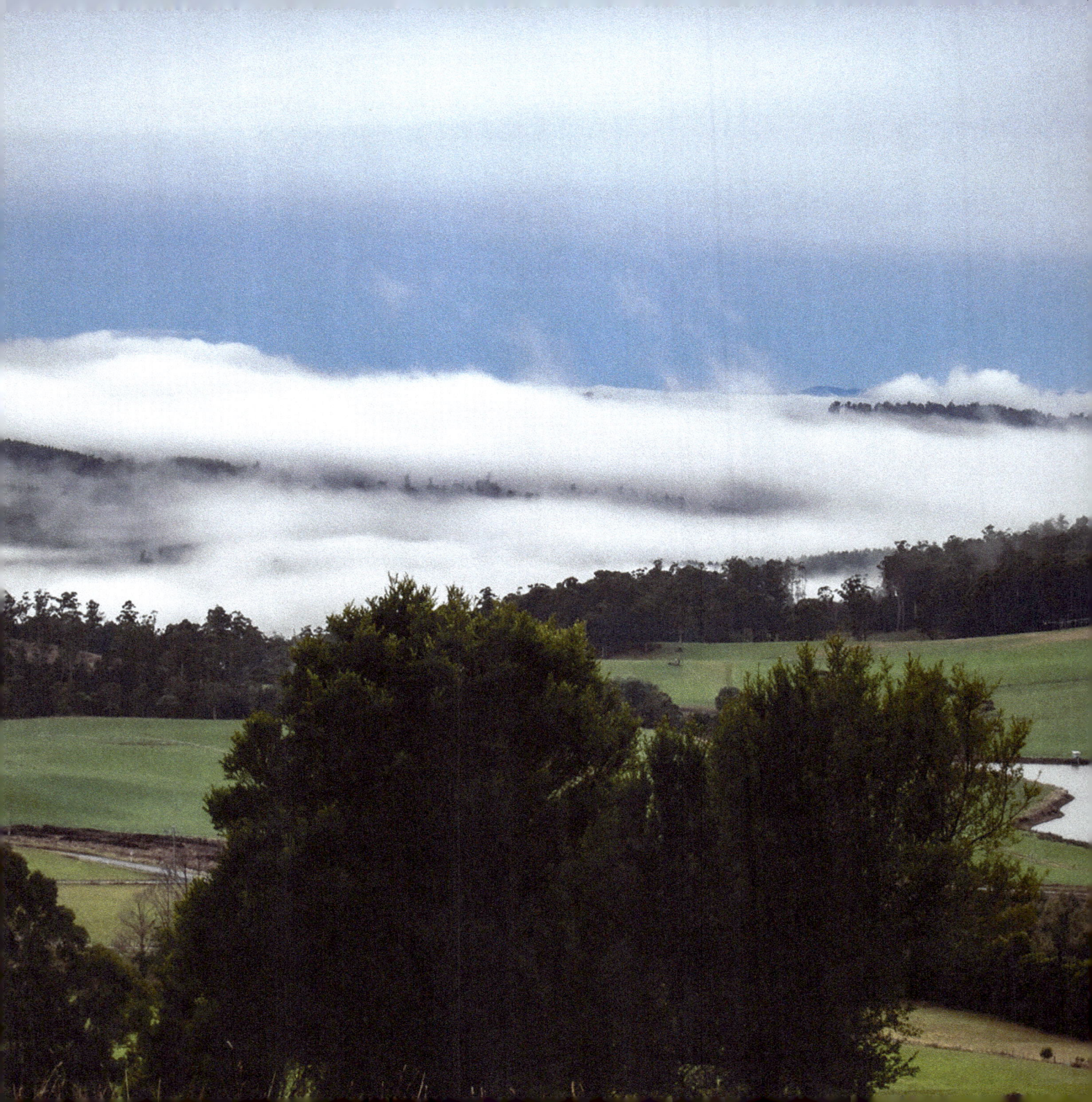

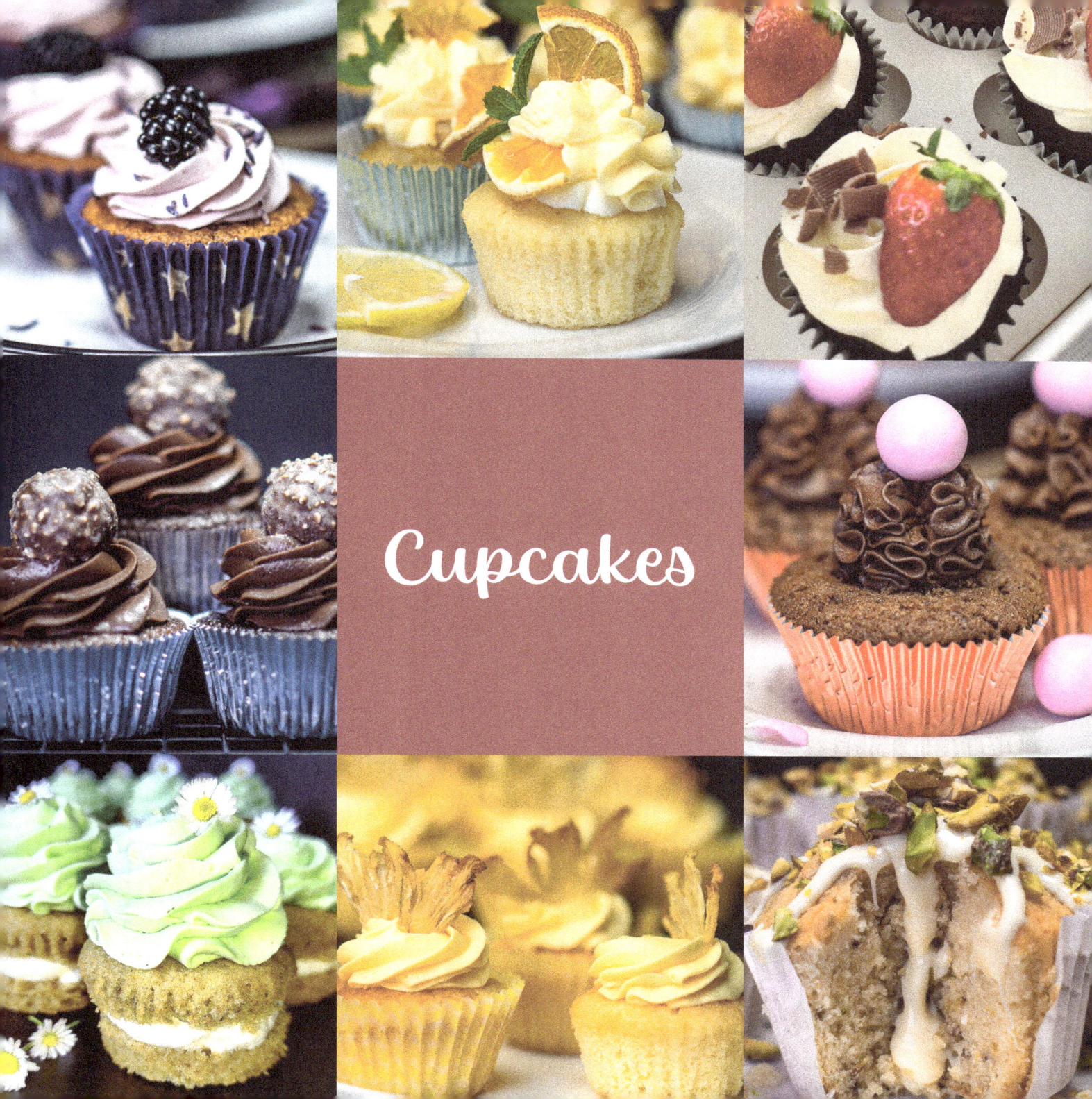
Cupcakes

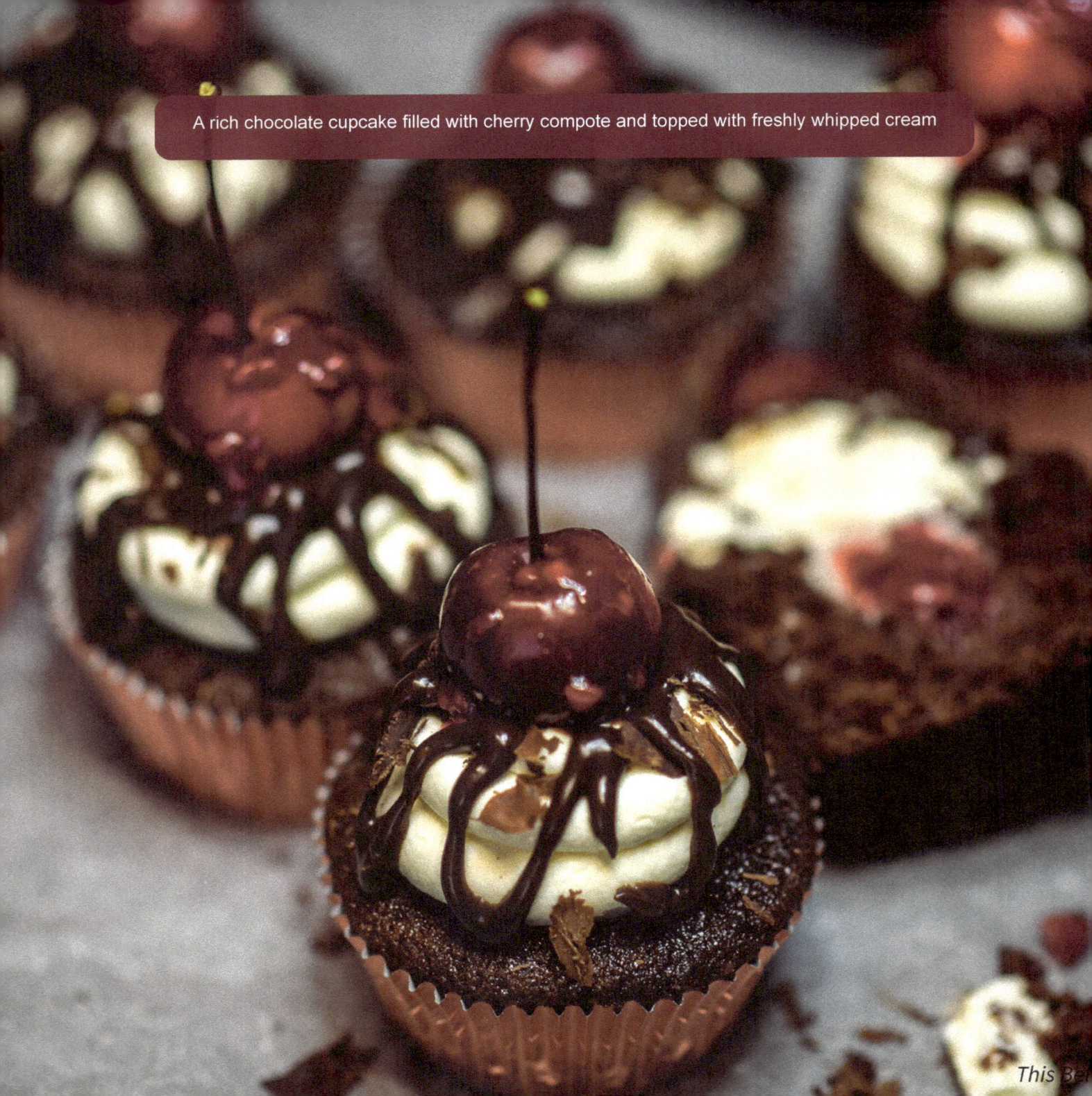
A rich chocolate cupcake filled with cherry compote and topped with freshly whipped cream

RICH BLACK FOREST CUPCAKES

Ingredients

150g (1 cup) cake flour
25g (¼ cup) Dutch cocoa powder
1 tsp espresso powder
1 ½ tsp baking powder
½ tsp salt
113g (½ cup) unsalted butter - *melted*
2 tbsp vegetable oil
200g granulated sugar
2 large eggs - *room temperature*
½ tsp vanilla extract
125ml (½ cup) whole milk

Cherry compote
1 bottle pitted morello cherries
2 tbsp granulated sugar
2 tbsp cornstarch
1 tbsp of cherry liquor (Kirsch) or just lemon juice

Whipped cream
500ml (2 cups) thickened cream
6 tbsp powdered sugar
1 tbsp milk powder
½ tsp vanilla extract

Top with
Fresh cherries
Dark chocolate shavings - *use vegetable peeler*

Method

Preparation for cherry syrup
1. Drain cherries, reserving liquid
2. Mix ¼ cup of cherry juice with corn flour to make a slurry. Set aside

Making the cherry compote
3. Using a medium pot on medium-low heat, add sugar and 1/3 cup of cherry juice until sugar dissolved
4. Add corn flour slurry, simmer until mixture thickens to a thin syrup.
5. Turn off heat, stir in cherry liquor or lemon juice.
6. Pour syrup over the drained cherries and allow to cool
7. Store leftover syrup in the fridge for future use

Making chocolate cupcakes
8. Preheat oven to 160° fan forced. Line a 12-cup pan with liners
9. Whisk flour, cocoa, espresso powder, baking powder and salt.
10. In another bowl, whisk butter, oil, eggs, sugar and vanilla
11. Stir in half of the flour mix, add milk, then the remaining flour. Mix until fully combined (don't over mix)
12. Fill liners halfway with batter
13. Bake at 160°C for 20-22 minutes or until cake tester comes out clean.
14. Let cupcakes cool completely before frosting and filling.

Preparing the whipped cream
15. Using an electric mixer whip cream, icing sugar, milk powder and vanilla to stiff peaks.

Assembly
16. Remove the centre of the cupcakes with an apple corer, set aside.
17. Fill with cherry compote and place the cut outs on top.
18. Pipe whipped cream, drizzle on chocolate ganache (pg # 109), sprinkle on chocolate shavings, add a cherry on top

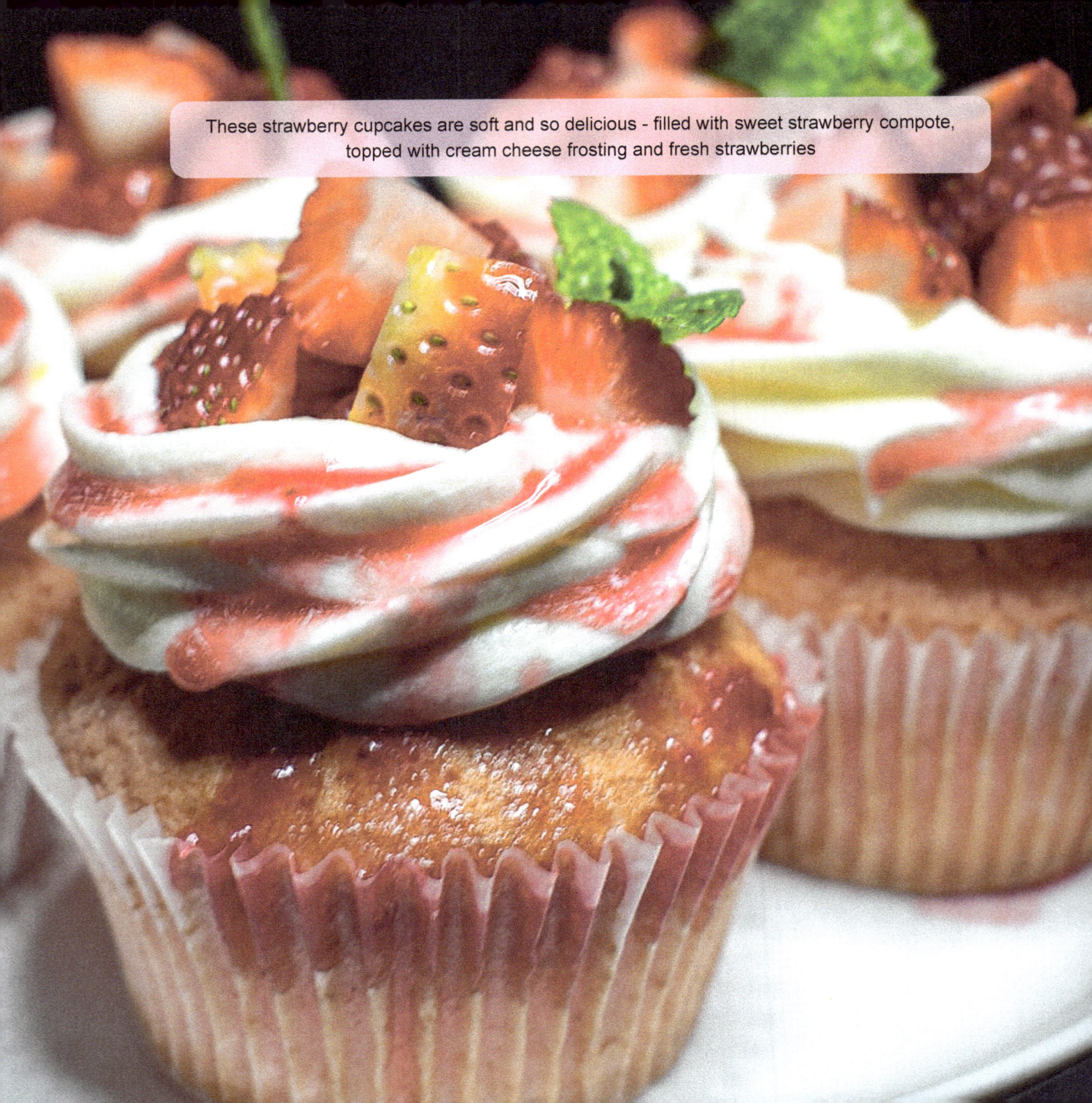
These strawberry cupcakes are soft and so delicious - filled with sweet strawberry compote, topped with cream cheese frosting and fresh strawberries

STRAWBERRY CREAM CHEESE CUPCAKES

Ingredients

Cupcakes

225g (1½ cups) cake flour
1 tsp baking powder
¼ tsp baking soda
¼ tsp salt
56g (¼ cup) unsalted butter - *at room temperature*
60ml (¼ cup) vegetable oil
220g (1 cup) granulated sugar
2 large eggs - *at room temperature*
1 tsp vanilla extract
125ml (½ cup) milk - *at room temperature*
1 drop strawberry flavour (I use Roberts)

Cream cheese frosting

250g cream cheese (I use Philadelphia) - *at room temperature*
113g (½ cup) unsalted butter - *at room temperature*
213g (1⅓ cup) powdered sugar - *sifted*
1½ tsp vanilla extract

Method

1. Preheat oven to 170°C fan forced. Line a 12-cup pan with paper liners.
2. In a large bowl, sift together the flour, baking powder, baking soda and salt, set aside
3. Using an electric mixer, beat the butter with the granulated sugar and oil on medium speed for about 1 minute, until creamy and fluffy.
4. Add the eggs, one at a time, mixing each egg until combined before adding the next. Add strawberry flavour, vanilla and mix
5. Add one third of the dry ingredient mixture. Mix on low speed until incorporated.
6. Add half of milk and mix to combine
7. Add another third of dry ingredients and mix and follow with the remaining milk
8. Lastly add the remainder of the dry ingredient and fold with a spatula.
9. Divide the batter evenly among the cupcake liners, filling each about two thirds full.
10. Bake for 18 minutes. Let the cupcakes cool before filling and frosting.

Cream cheese frosting

11. Using an electric mixer, mix the cream cheese and butter on medium/high for 4 minutes, until very fluffy and light in colour
12. Add the sifted powdered sugar and mix on low speed until combined, increase the speed to medium high and beat for another minute. Add vanilla and mix until combined.

Assembly

13. Remove the centre of each cupcake with an apple corer,
14. Add the strawberry compote filling into each cupcake
15. Place the cream cheese frosting in a piping bag, fitted with 1M piping tip. Pipe a tall ring around the edge of the cupcakes, leaving a hole in the middle, spoon some more strawberry compote into the middle of the frosting ring. Top with fresh strawberry.

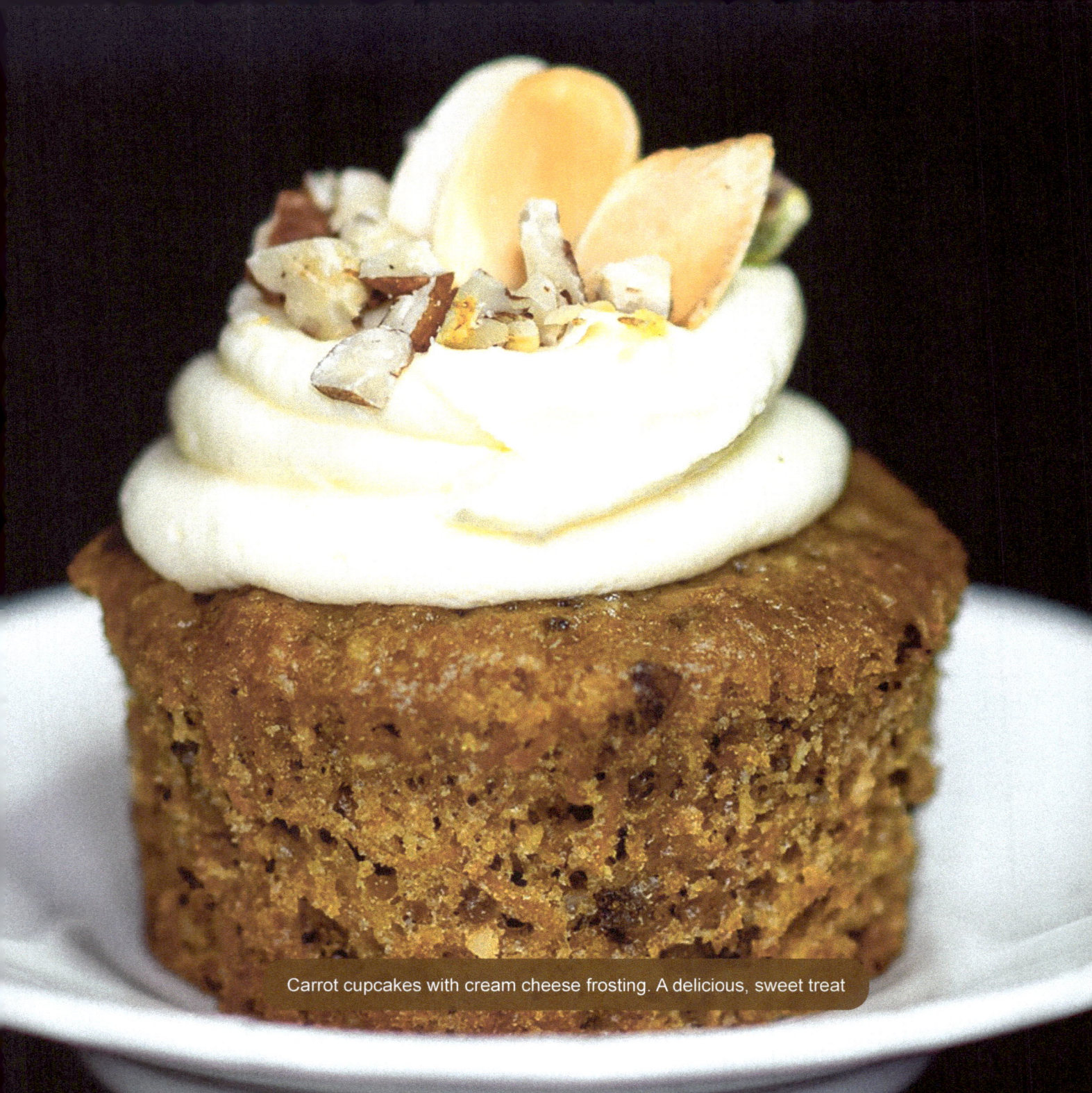
Carrot cupcakes with cream cheese frosting. A delicious, sweet treat

CARROT CUPCAKES

Ingredients

150g (1 cup) all-purpose flour
110g (½ cup) granulated sugar
110g (½ cup) brown sugar
¾ tsp baking soda
½ tsp baking powder
½ tsp salt
1 tsp ground cinnamon
¼ tsp nutmeg
63ml (¼ cup) crushed pineapple fruit, or juice
180ml (¾ cup + 1 tbsp) vegetable oil
2 large eggs - *at room temperature*
1½ tsp vanilla extract
2 tbsp milk
180g grated carrot - *about 3 big carrots*
60g chopped walnuts or pecans - *optional*

Cream cheese frosting

113g (½ cup) unsalted butter - *softened*
250g cream cheese – *Philadelphia recommended*
1 tsp vanilla extract
¼ tsp salt
330g (1½ cups) sugar

Method

1. Preheat oven to 170°C fan-forced and line a 12 cupcakes pan with paper liners.

2. In a bowl, whisk flour, sugar, baking powder, baking soda, salt cinnamon and nutmeg.

3. Stir in vegetable oil. Add eggs, one at a time and mix until well combined.

4. Add vanilla extract, pineapple juice and milk.

5. Add carrot and nuts and stir until combined.

6. Evenly divide batter into cupcake liners, filling each ¾ full. Transfer to oven and bake on 170°C for 20 minutes, or until skewer inserted in the centre comes out clean.

7. Allow to cool completely before decorating with cream cheese frosting.

Cream cheese frosting

8. Combine butter and cream cheese in a bowl with an electric mixer. Beat until creamy and lump free. Add vanilla extract and salt, stir well. With mixer on low, gradually add powdered sugar and mix until completely combined.

9. Add frosting to the cupcakes once they are completely cooled.

10. Garnish with roasted pecans or walnuts.

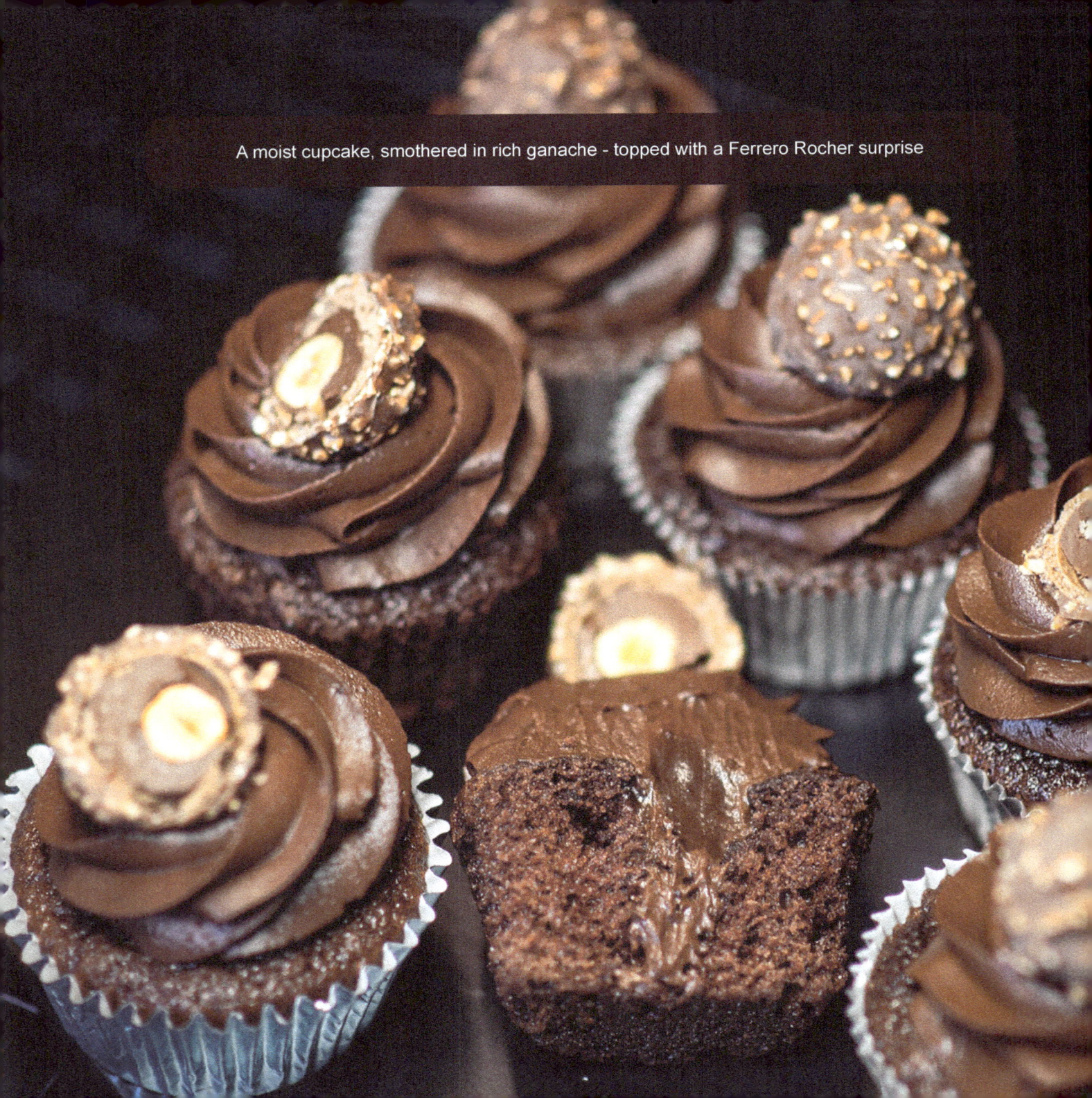
A moist cupcake, smothered in rich ganache - topped with a Ferrero Rocher surprise

CHOCOLATE GANACHE CUPCAKES

Ingredients

150g (1 cup) all-purpose flour
38g (¼ cup + 2 tbsp) cocoa powder
½ tsp baking soda
½ tsp baking powder
220g (1 cup) caster sugar
¼ tsp salt
110ml (½ cup) coffee - cooled
113ml (½ cup) butter milk - *(milk + 1 tsp white vinegar/sour cream/yogurt)*
50ml (¼ cup) vegetable oil
2 egg - *at room temperature*
1 tsp vanilla extract
Chocolate ganache (please see page 109)

Method

1. Brew the coffee and let it cool to room temperature.
2. Preheat oven to 170°C fan forced
3. Line a 12-cup standard size muffin pan with cupcake liners and set aside.
4. In a large mixing bowl, whisk together cooled coffee, buttermilk, oil, eggs and vanilla until thoroughly combined.
5. Sift the flour, cocoa powder, baking soda, baking powder in another bowl. Add salt and sugar and whisk until evenly distributed.
6. Add the flour mixture to the wet ingredients mixture and stir until a smooth batter forms.
7. Divide the batter evenly into 12 muffin cups, using a large cookie scoop. Bake for 17- 19 minutes until skewer inserted in the middle of the cupcakes comes out clean.
8. Allow the cupcakes to cool in the pan for 10 minutes until cool to touch. Remove them from the pan and place them on wire rack to cool completely.
9. Fill the piping bag fitted with an open stars piping tip (1m) and pipe swirls of chocolate ganache on the top of cupcakes. Enjoy

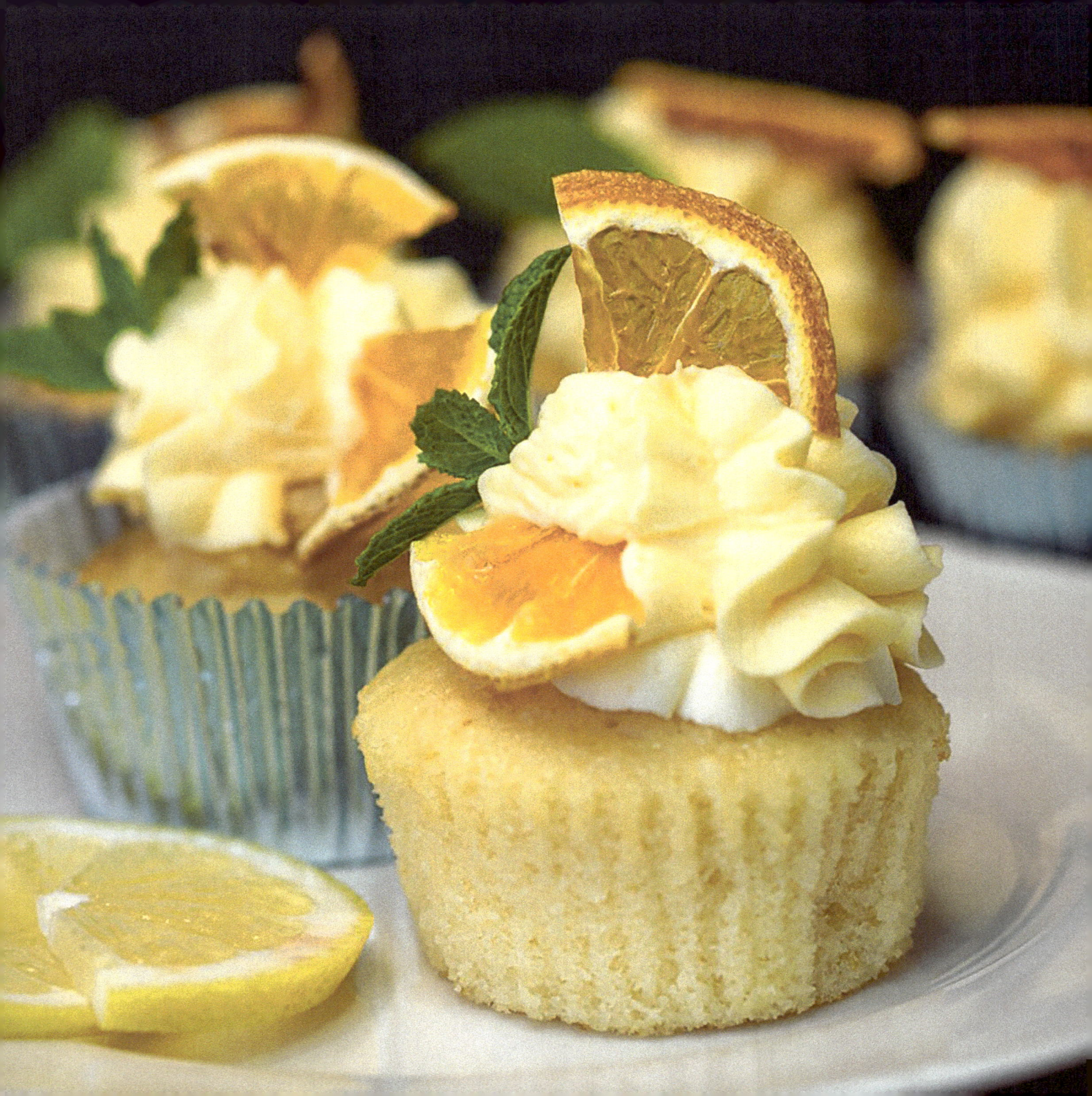

LEMON CUPCAKES

Citrusy lemon, topped with a zesty slice of dried orange

Ingredients

Frosting

200g (1⅓ cups) all-purpose flour
220g (1 cup) caster sugar
2 tbsp lemon zest (zest of 2 lemons)
¼ tsp baking soda
1½ tsp baking powder
¼ tsp salt
2 eggs - room temperature
125ml (½ cup) sour cream/yogurt - *room temperature*
63ml milk (¼ cup)- *room temperature*
60ml (¼ cup) lemon juice

The Buttercream

225g (1 cup) unsalted butter - *softened*
320g (2 cup) icing sugar
¼ tsp salt
Lemon juice - *from 1 lemon*
2 tbsp lemon zest

Method

1. Preheat oven to 170 °C fan forced. Line a 12-hole cupcake pan with paper cases
2. Using food processor, mix sugar and lemon zest, pulse until the mix is a pale yellow colour.
3. In a large bowl, sift the flour, baking soda, baking powder and salt. Whisk together, set aside.
4. In a medium bowl whisk together eggs, milk, melted butter, lemon juice, sour cream and sugar. Everything should be room temperature.
5. Add the wet ingredients to the dry mixture and mix until just combined – do not over mix.
6. Fill cupcake papers evenly to ¾ full, bake for 18-20 minutes at 170 °C, or until the skewer inserted comes up clean. Allow to cool for 5 minutes and transfer to a wire rack until completely cool.

Lemon Buttercream

7. Cream the butter, salt and zest then gradually sift in the icing sugar, in a few batches, mixing well
8. Scrape the bowl down and pour in lemon juice while mixing on low speed until all is incorporated and creamy.

Assembly

9. Cut the middle out of the cooled cupcakes with an apple corer
10. Nest the cupcakes with lemon curd (see page 108 for lemon curd recipe)
11. Place the cut out back on top, piping with lemon butter cream, and garnish with a slice of dried orange.

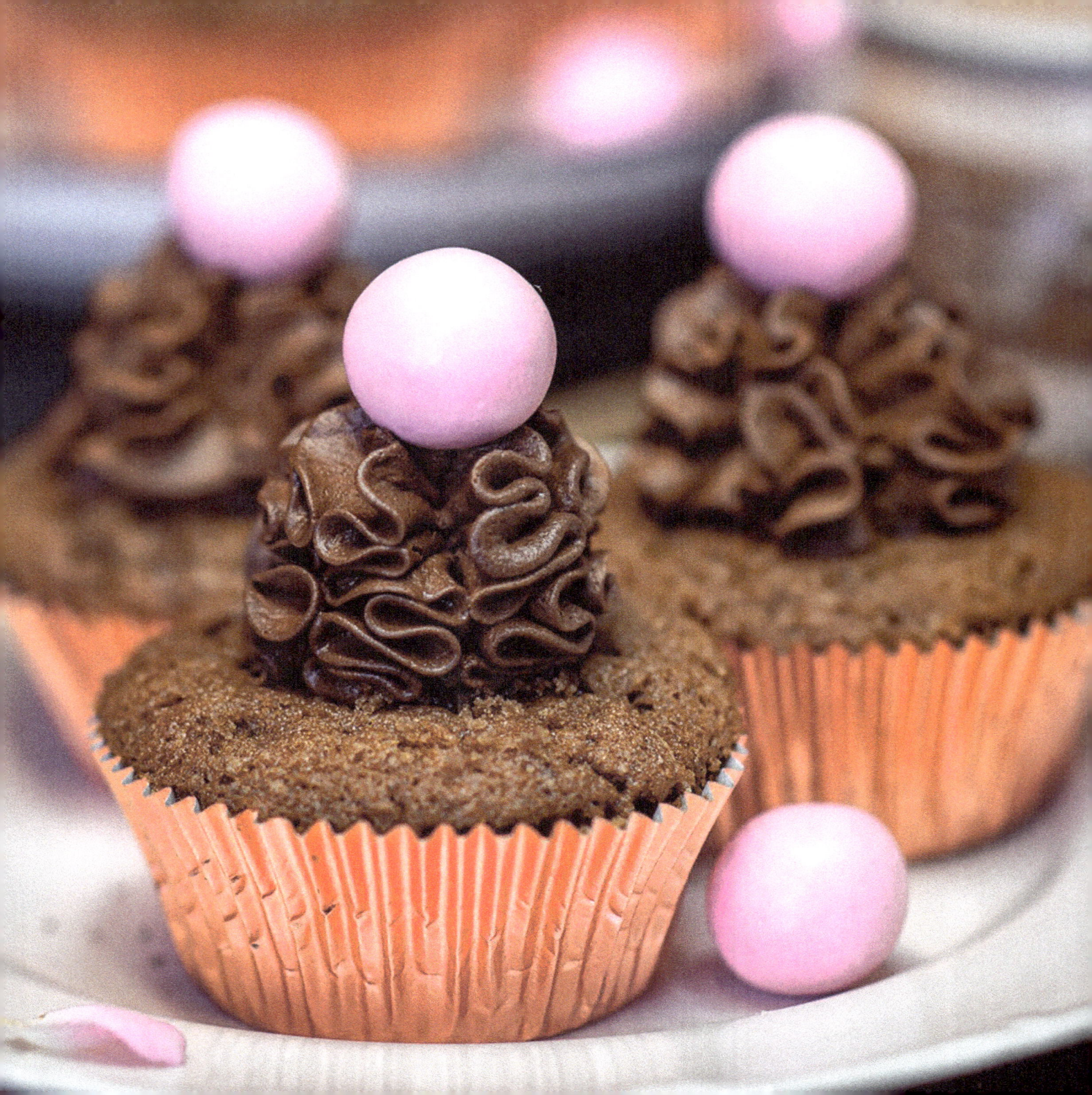

MOCHA CUPCAKES

These mocha cupcakes the perfect balance of coffee and espresso infused, light in the chocolate and topped with espresso frosting

Ingredients

Cupcakes

150g (1 cup) all-purpose flour
25g (¼ cup) cocoa powder
80g (½ cup) granulated sugar
110g (½ cup) light brown sugar
1 tsp baking powder
½ tsp baking soda
¼ tsp salt
125ml (½ cup) hot water - *for brewing the espresso powder*
1½ tsp espresso powder
125ml milk (½ cup) - at room temperature
113g (½ cup) unsalted butter – *at room temperature*
2 eggs - *at room temperature*
1 tsp vanilla extract

Espresso Frosting

450g (2 cups) unsalted butter - *at room temperature*
640g (4 cups) powdered sugar
1½ tsp vanilla extract
20ml espresso

Method

1. Preheat oven to 170°C fan forced. Line a standard size cupcakes tin with paper liners
2. In a measuring cup, whisk the espresso powder in the hot water until completely dissolved. Add milk and vanilla, set aside
3. In large bowl, whisk together the flour, cocoa powder, baking powder, baking soda, salt
4. In another bowl, using an electric mixer on medium speed, beat butter and both sugars until fluffy. Add eggs, one at the time and beat until combined. Reduce the mixer speed to low and add the flour mixture in three separate additions. Give the batter a final stir using a spatula, until the batter is all incorporated.
5. Fill each cupcake liner about two thirds full of batter. Bake for 18 minutes or until springs back when touched. Cool completely before frosting.

Making the frosting

6. In a small bowl, whisk the espresso and vanilla until dissolved, set aside
7. Whip the butter on medium, high speed with stand mixer until pale. Reduce the mixer speed to low and add the powdered sugar a little at a time, once all the powdered sugar has been added. Scrape the sides of the bowl and whip until fluffy.
8. Add the espresso and vanilla mixture and continue mixer until completely incorporated.
9. Frost the cupcakes as desired.

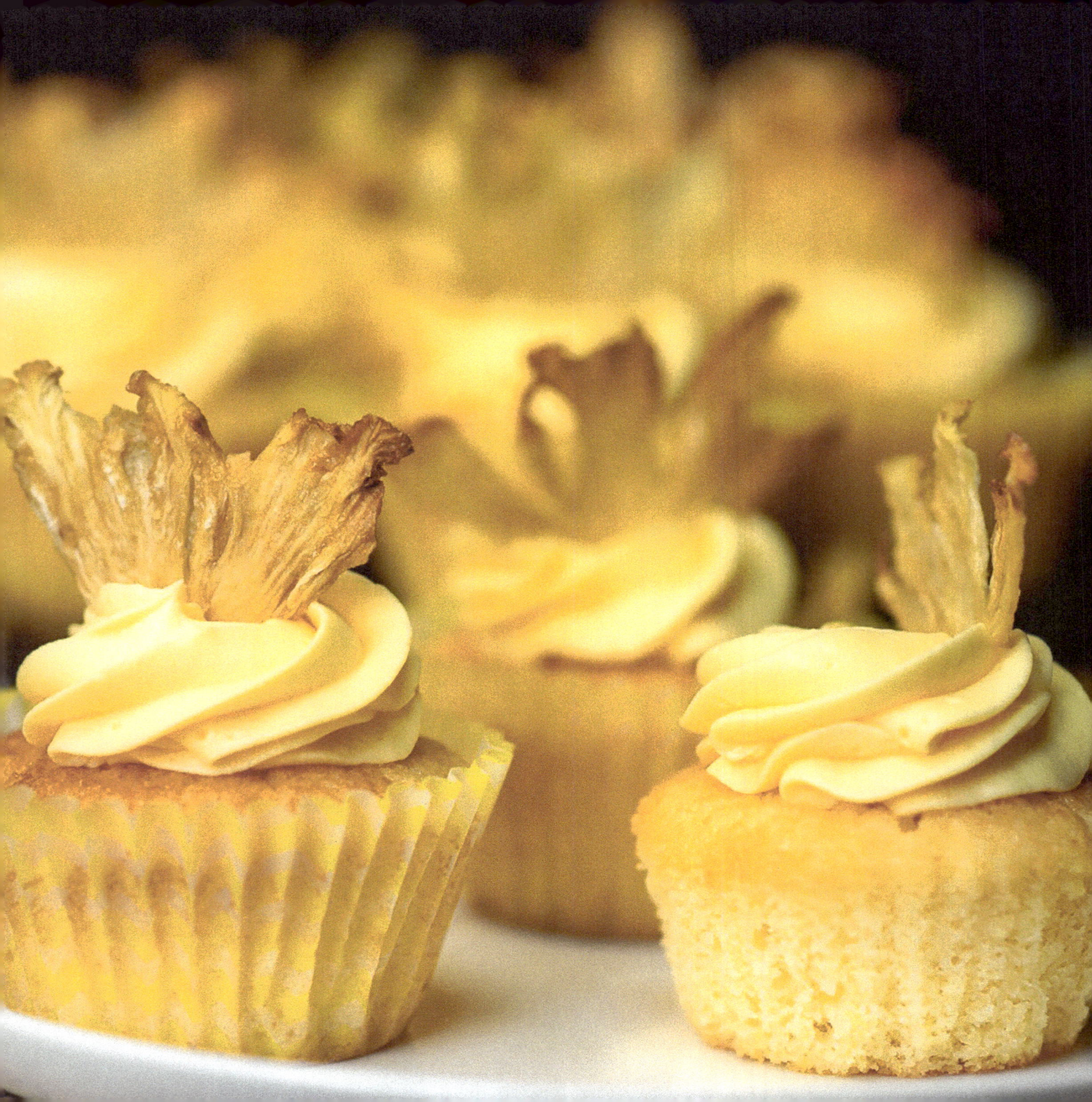

PINEAPPLE CUPCAKES

Delicious buttery cupcakes bursting with pineapple flavour and swirled with pineapple frosting

Ingredients

188g (1¼ cups) all-purpose flour
55g (¼ cup) light brown sugar
110g (½ cup) granulated sugar
1 tsp baking powder
¼ tsp salt
113g (½ cup) unsalted butter - *softened*
2 large eggs – *at room temperature*
250g crushed pineapple - *undrained*
1 tsp vanilla extract

Frosting

170g (¾ cup) unsalted butter - *softened* at room temperature
266g (1 ⅔ cup) soft icing sugar - *sifted*
1 tsp vanilla extract
⅛ tsp salt
45g (3 tbsp) thickened cream – *at room temperature*
¼ tsp pineapple flavouring

Garnish

Dried pineapple

Method

1. Preheat oven to 170°C fan-forced and line a 12 cupcakes pan with paper liners.
2. In a medium sized mixing bowl, combine and whisk the flour, baking powder and salt.
3. In separate mixing bowl beat the butter until creamy. Add sugar and continue beating. Set the mixer to low and add vanilla, then beat in the eggs one at a time, mixing well
4. In a separate mixing bowl, beat the crushed pineapple to juice, add the butter mixture and then fold in the flour mixture until combined.
5. Divide evenly into cupcake liners, filling each ¾ full. Transfer to oven and bake on 170°C for 18-20 minutes, or until skewer inserted in the centre comes out clean.
6. Allow the cupcakes to cool for 5 minutes before transferring to a wire rack to cool completely. Top with pineapple frosting.

Making the frosting

7. Using a stand mixer, fitted with the paddle attachment, beat the buttercream on medium to high speed until creamy and pale in colour – approximately 5 minutes
8. Add half of soft icing sugar, beat on low speed just until the sugar is fully combined, then increase the speed to medium/high and beat until well incorporated – approximately 3 minutes
9. Add vanilla, pineapple flavouring, salt, thickened cream and the remaining soft icing sugar and beat together until a soft and spreadable consistency.

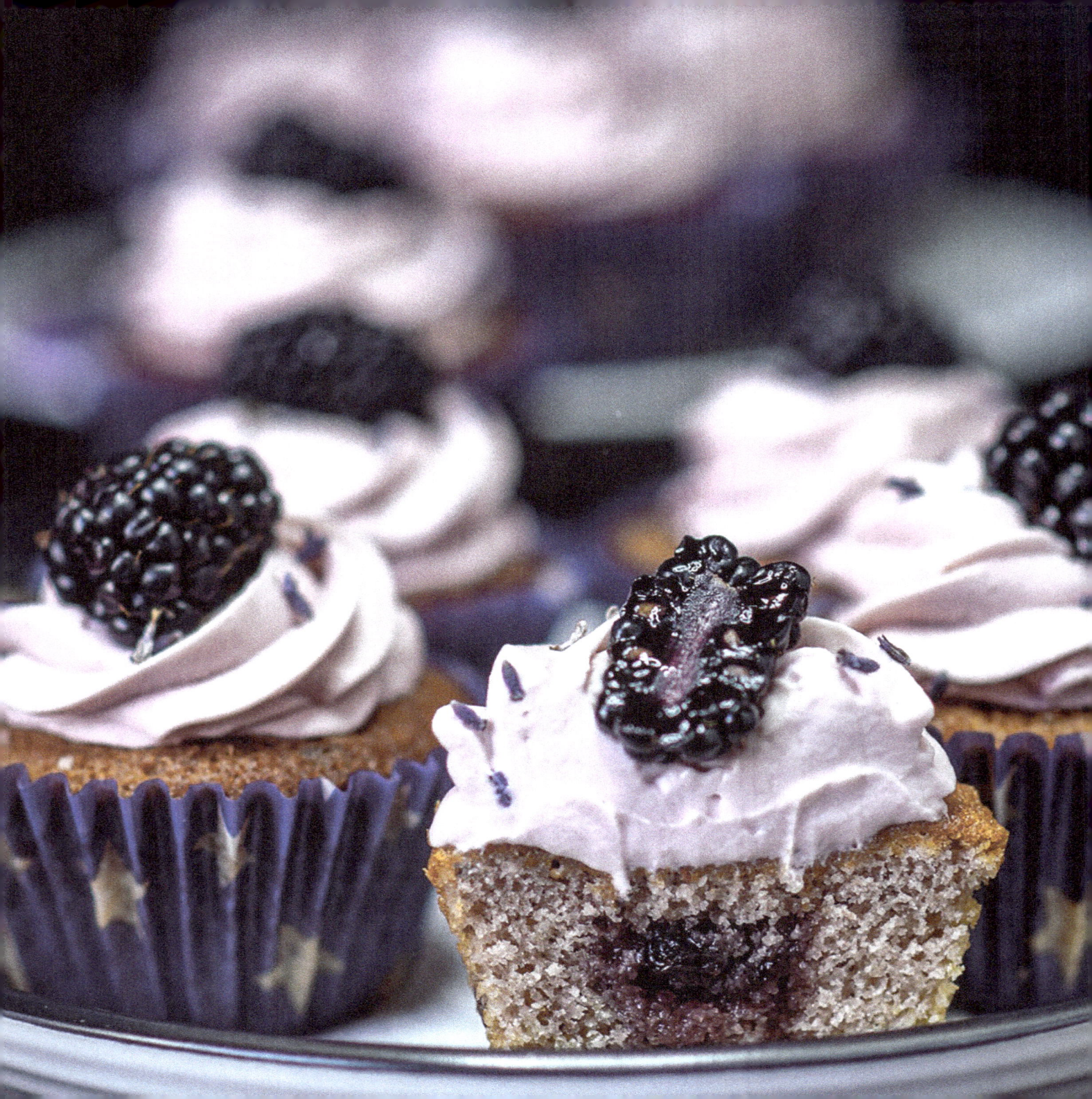

LAVENDER CUPCAKES

Lavender desserts have always felt so fancy to me. By infusing dried lavender with milk it gives these cupcakes a light floral flavour that pairs beautifully with tangy blackberry lavender jam.

Ingredients

Lavender infused milk

125ml (½ cup) milk
2 tsp dried lavender
1 drop of purple food gel for the lavender cupcakes

Blackberry lavender jam

450g (16 oz) blackberries - *fresh or frozen*
145g (⅔ cup) granulated sugar
2 tsp lemon juice
½ tsp dried lavender

Lavender butter cream

225g (1 cup) unsalted butter - *at room temperature*
400g (2½ cups) soft icing sugar
1 drop purple colouring
2 tsp thickened cream

Lavender cupcakes

113g (½ cup) unsalted butter - *melted*
220g (1 cup) granulated sugar
2 large eggs – *room temperature*
1 tsp vanilla extract
225g (1½ cups) cake flour
1½ tsp baking powder
¼ tsp salt

Method

Lavender Infused Milk

1. Cook milk in a small sauce pan on low heat. Add dried lavender for 2 minutes. Allow to cool and add the purple colour.

Blackberry lavender jam

2. Add all of the ingredients to a large saucepan, heating on medium low heat. Allow jam simmer for 15 to 20 minutes, stirring frequently until thickened.

Cupcakes

5. Preheat oven to 160°C fan-forced and line a 12 cupcakes pan with paper liners.

6. Whisk cake flour, baking powder and salt in a large bowl

7. In a separate bowl, whisk the melted butter, sugar, eggs and vanilla until combined

8. Stir in half of the flour mixture, then stir in the lavender milk. Mix until fluffy and combined - the batter will be thin. Pour into cupcake liners - half way full

9. Bake for 20 to 22 minutes or until the cake tester comes out clean

10. Remove from the pan and allow to cool on a wire rack. Allow cupcakes to cool completely before filling and frosting

11. Remove the centre of each cupcake with a cupcake corer. Fill with 2 tsp of cooled blackberry jam

Lavender Buttercream

13. In a stand mixer fitted with the paddle attachment, cream together the softened butter and icing sugar until smooth and creamy

14. Add the purple colouring food and thickened cream until light and fluffy

15. Frost the cooled cupcakes.

Decorating

17. Fill the piping bag fitted with open star piping tip (1m) and pipe swirls of lavender butter cream on top of the cake

18. Sprinkle with dried lavender and/or add a blackberry - as desired.

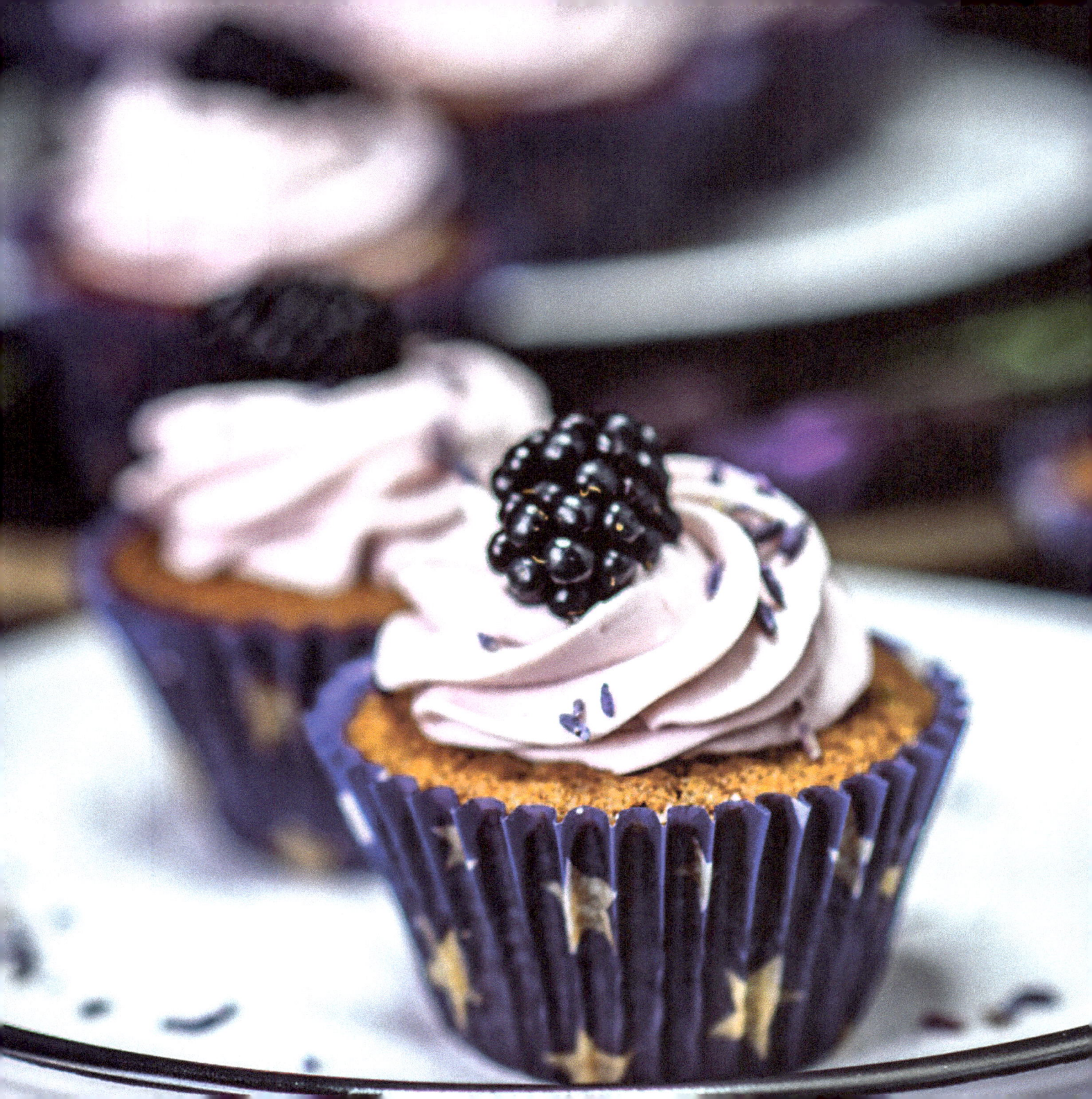

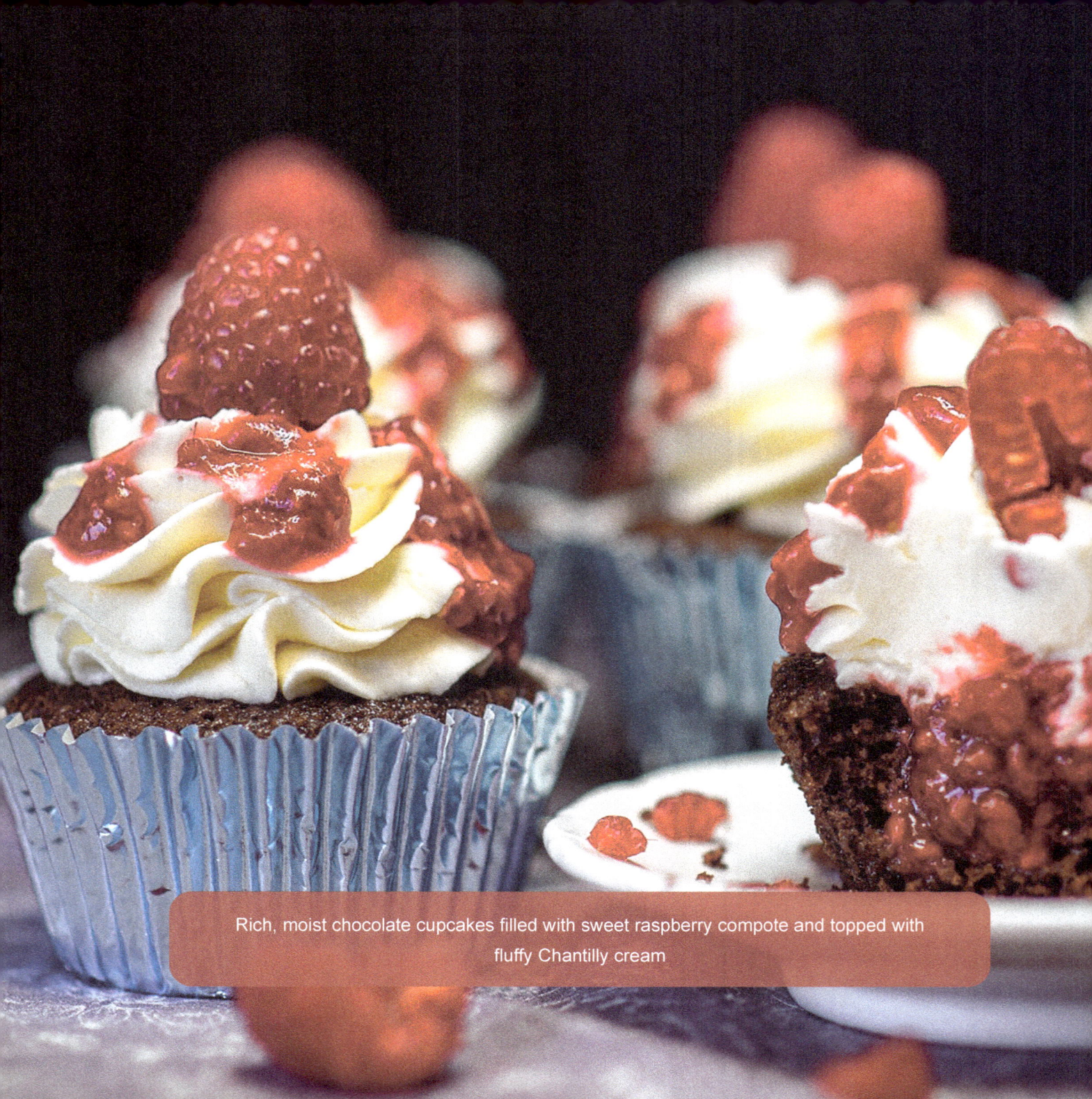

Rich, moist chocolate cupcakes filled with sweet raspberry compote and topped with fluffy Chantilly cream

CHANTILLY DREAM CUPCAKES WITH RASPBERRY COMPOTE

Ingredients

Cupcakes
263g (1¾ cups) all-purpose flour
550g (1½ cups) sugar
75g (¾ cup) Dutch cocoa powder
1½ tsp baking powder
1½ tsp baking soda
½ tsp salt
2 large eggs - at room temperature
2 tsp Vanilla extract
250ml (1 cup) milk
120ml (½ cup) vegetable oil
30 ml espresso
250ml (1 cup) boiling water

Raspberry buttercream frosting
150g raspberries (frozen or fresh)
3 tbsp white sugar
1 tbsp corn starch - *mixed with 3 tbsp water*

Chantilly Cream Topping
375ml (1½ cups) thickened cream
6 tbsp soft icing sugar
1 tsp vanilla extract
2 tbsp milk powder

Method

Cupcakes
1. Preheat oven to 160°C fan forced. Line a muffin tin with paper cupcakes liners
2. In a small bowl, whisk together eggs, oil, milk, vanilla extract and espresso
3. In a small bowl sift flour, cocoa powder, baking powder, baking soda, sugar and salt set aside
4. Gently add the dry ingredient to the wet ingredients mixing until just combined – do not over mix, as it can lead to dense cupcakes. The add the hot water (being careful as you can expect the batter to be quite runny).
5. Divide the batter evenly into the cupcake liners, filling each to about ¾ full
6. Bake for about 20 minutes or until a skewer inserted into the centre comes out clean. Remove from the oven and allow to cool.

Raspberry compote
7. Combine raspberries and sugar in a saucepan
8. Cook over medium heat, stirring occasionally until bubbling, then add cornstarch slurry and remove from the heat. Wait until completely cool.

Chantilly Cream
9. In a large mixing bowl, combine the thickened cream, powdered sugar, milk powder and vanilla extract.
10. Beat with an electric mixer on medium high speed until stiff peaks form - about 2-3 minutes

Decorating
11. Core the hole in the centre of each cupcake and fill with raspberry compote
12. Pipe a swirl of Chantilly cream on top using an M1 tip
13. Garnish with a fresh raspberry.

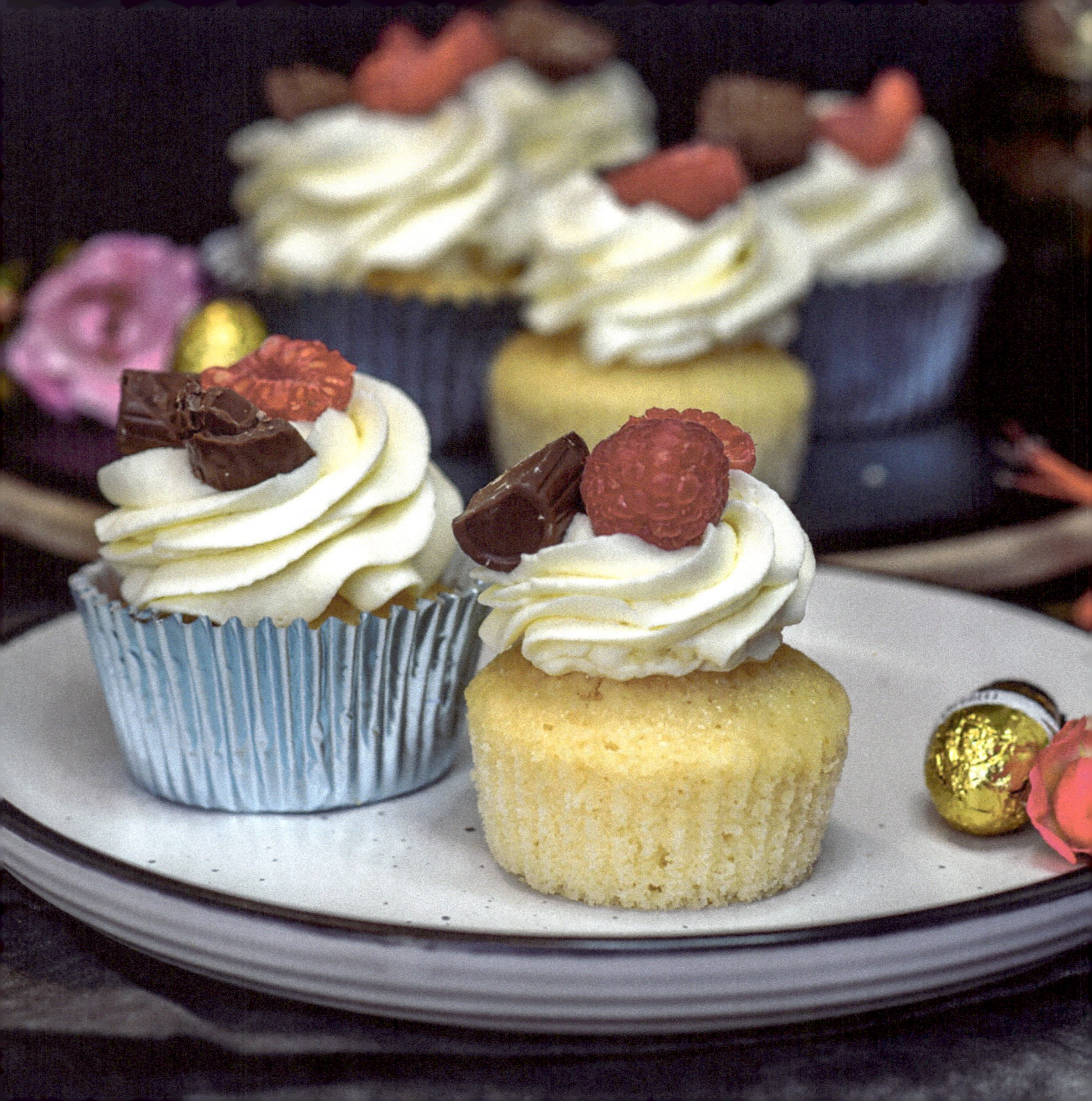

CHANTILLY EASTER BITES

Ingredients

100g (⅔ cup) cup self-raising flour - *sifted*
110g (½ cup) cup caster superfine sugar
113g (½ cup) butter - *softened*
2 large eggs - *at room temperature*
1 tsp vanilla extract

For decorating

500ml (2 cups) thickened cream
5 tsp powdered sugar
1 tsp vanilla extract
2 tbsp milk powder
12 chocolate mini eggs
Raspberries

Method

1. Preheat the oven for 160° and line a 12 hole cupcake tin with paper cases

2. Combine butter and sugar. Whisk until creamy. Add eggs and vanilla extract. Then slowly add self-raising flour. Don't over mix- just combine.

3. Divide the mixture into the paper cases and bake for 17-20 minutes

4. Test with a wooden toothpick. If it comes out clean, the cupcakes are done.

5. Transfer the cupcakes to a wire rack and allow to cool completely

6. Blend thickened cream, icing sugar, milk powder and vanilla at high speed for 3 to 5 minutes, or until stiff peaks form.

Decorating

7. Spoon the chantilly cream into a piping bag, fitted with a large star nozzle, and pipe a swirl of frosting on top of the cupcakes, then top each one with raspberry and a mini chocolate Easter egg.

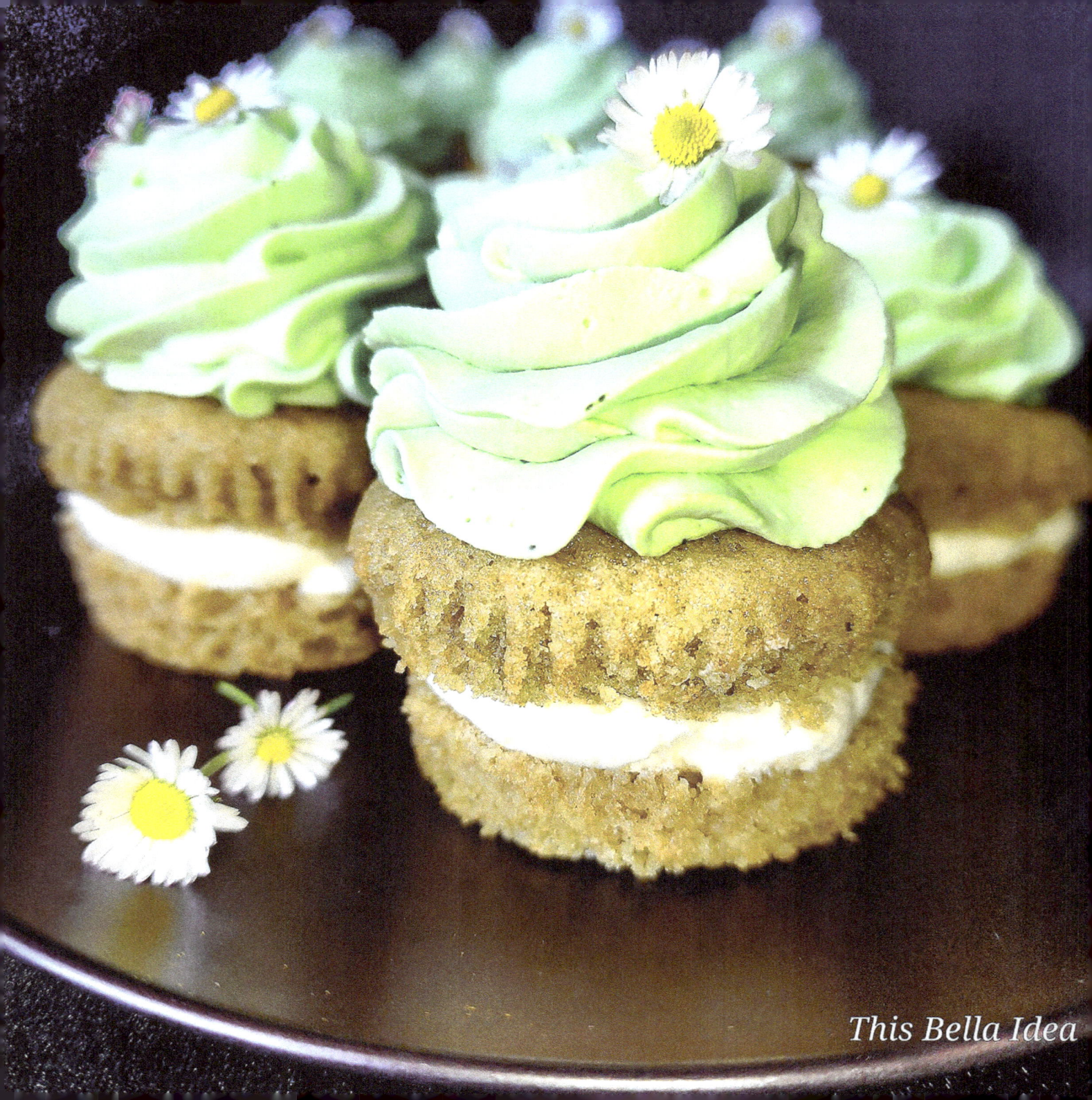

MATCHA GREEN TEA CUPCAKES

Ingredients

120ml (½ cup) whole milk

1 tsp loose green tea

113g (½ cup) unsalted butter - *softened*

145g (⅔ cup) caster sugar

2 large eggs - *at room temperature*

150g (1 cup) self-raising flour - *sifted*

¼ tsp baking powder

The filling

56g (¼ cup) unsalted butter - *softened*

160g (1 cup) soft icing sugar - *sifted*

40ml (⅙ cup) milk

The topping

¼ tsp loose green matcha tea

83ml (⅓ cup) boiling water

56g (¼ cup) unsalted butter - *softened*

160g (1 cup) soft icing sugar - *sifted*

Method

1. Preheat oven to 170 °C fan forced. Line a 12-hole muffin pan with paper cases
2. Put milk in a small saucepan and bring to boil. Add green tea leaves and infuse for 30 minutes.
3. Using the mixer, whisk the butter and caster sugar in a bowl until pale and creamy, gradually whisk the eggs until just combined. Pass the green tea milk through a sieve into the bowl, then discard the tea. Using a spatula, fold in the flour and baking powder until combined. Divide the mixture equally between the paper cases.
4. Bake for 18-20 minutes until a golden colour and cupcakes have risen fully. Transfer to a wire rack to cool completely.

Filling

5. Whisk the butter in a bowl until fluffy, gradually add half of the icing sugar, whisking until combined. Add the milk and remaining icing sugar and whisk until light and fluffy.

Topping

6. Put the green tea leaves into a jug, add 75ml boiling water and infuse for 5 minutes.
7. Put the butter into a bowl and whisk until fluffy, gradually add the icing sugar and whisk until combined
8. Pass the green tea through a sieve into the bowl. Continue to whisk until light and fluffy.

Assembly

9. Cut the cupcakes in half. Insert a round nozzle into a piping bag, then fill the bag with butter cream and pipe around the cupcakes.
10. For the top, insert a star nozzle into the piping bag, fill the piping bag with matcha butter cream, and pipe a swirl onto the top of each cupcake. Add a decoration of your choice.

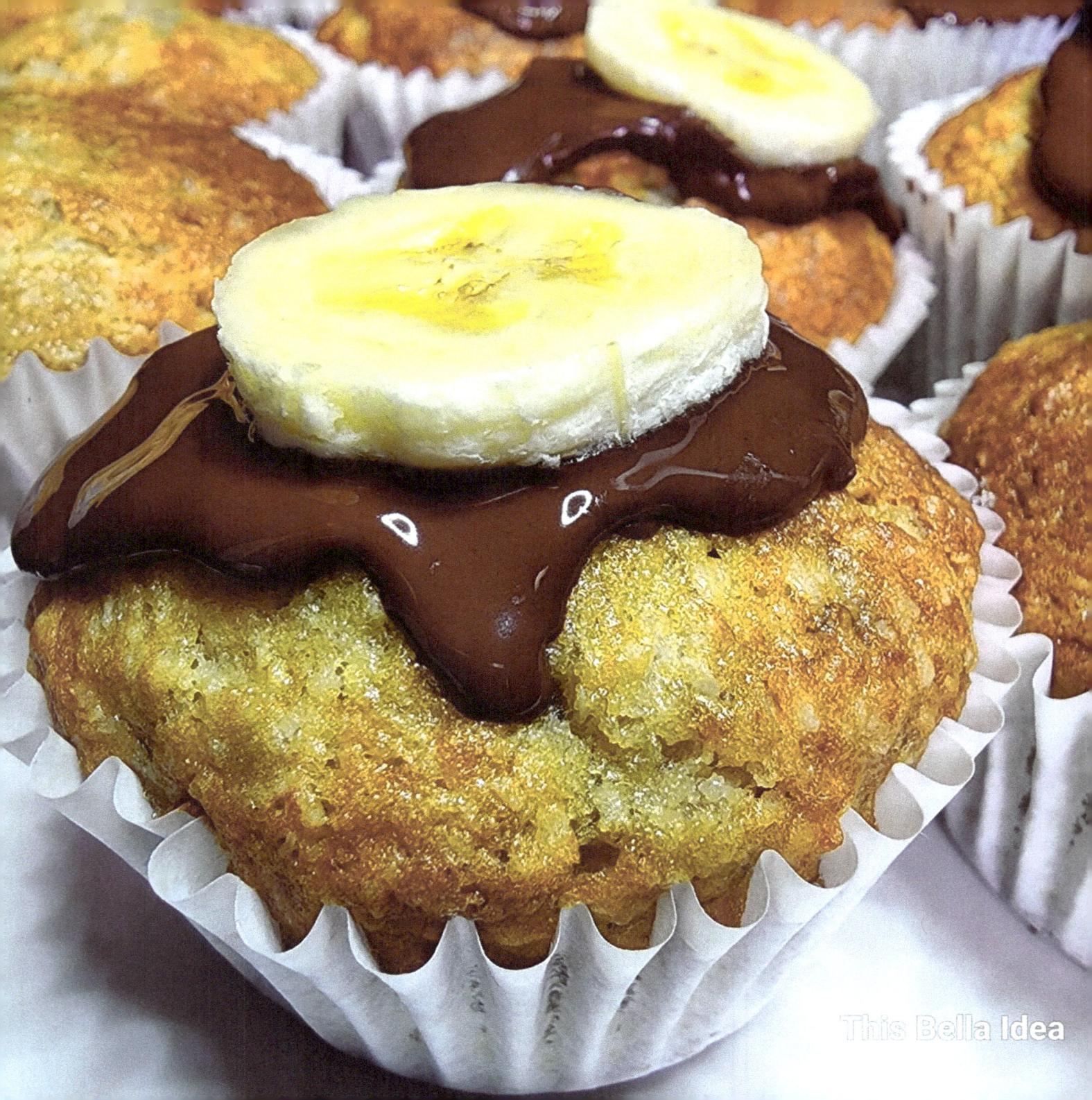

BANANA LOVE IN EVERY BITE

These delicious banana cupcakes are soft, buttery and spiced with cinnamon. You'll need 3 ripe bananas and a handful of basic kitchen ingredients.

Ingredients

350g mashed bananas - *approx. 3 large ripe bananas*
74g (⅓ cup) unsalted butter - *melted*
145g (⅔ cup) coconut sugar - *or light brown sugar*
1 large egg - *at room temperature*
1 tsp vanilla extract
2 tbsp milk - *at room temperature*
188g (1¼ cup) all-purpose flour
1 tsp baking soda
1 tsp baking powder
½ tsp salt
1 tsp ground cinnamon
¼ tsp ground nutmeg

Garnish
Chocolate bars
Banana slices

Method

1. Preheat oven to 180 °C fan forced. Line a 12-cup pan with paper liners.

2. Whisk the flour, baking powder, baking soda, salt, cinnamon and nutmeg together in a medium bowl, set aside.

3. In a large bowl, mash the bananas on medium speed. Beat or whisk in melted butter, brown sugar, egg, vanilla extract and milk.

4. Pour the dry ingredients into the wet ingredients, then beat or whisk until combined. If you are adding chocolate chips, fold them in now.

5. Spoon the batter into cupcake liners, filling them ¾ full.

6. Bake in 180 °C for 18 to 20 minutes or until skewer inserted into the centre comes out clean. Allow the cupcakes to cool for 3 minutes and then transfer to wire cooling rack to continue cooling.

7. Top warm banana cupcakes with a piece of chocolate and return to the oven until chocolate is melted

8. Remove from oven and finish with a slice of fresh banana

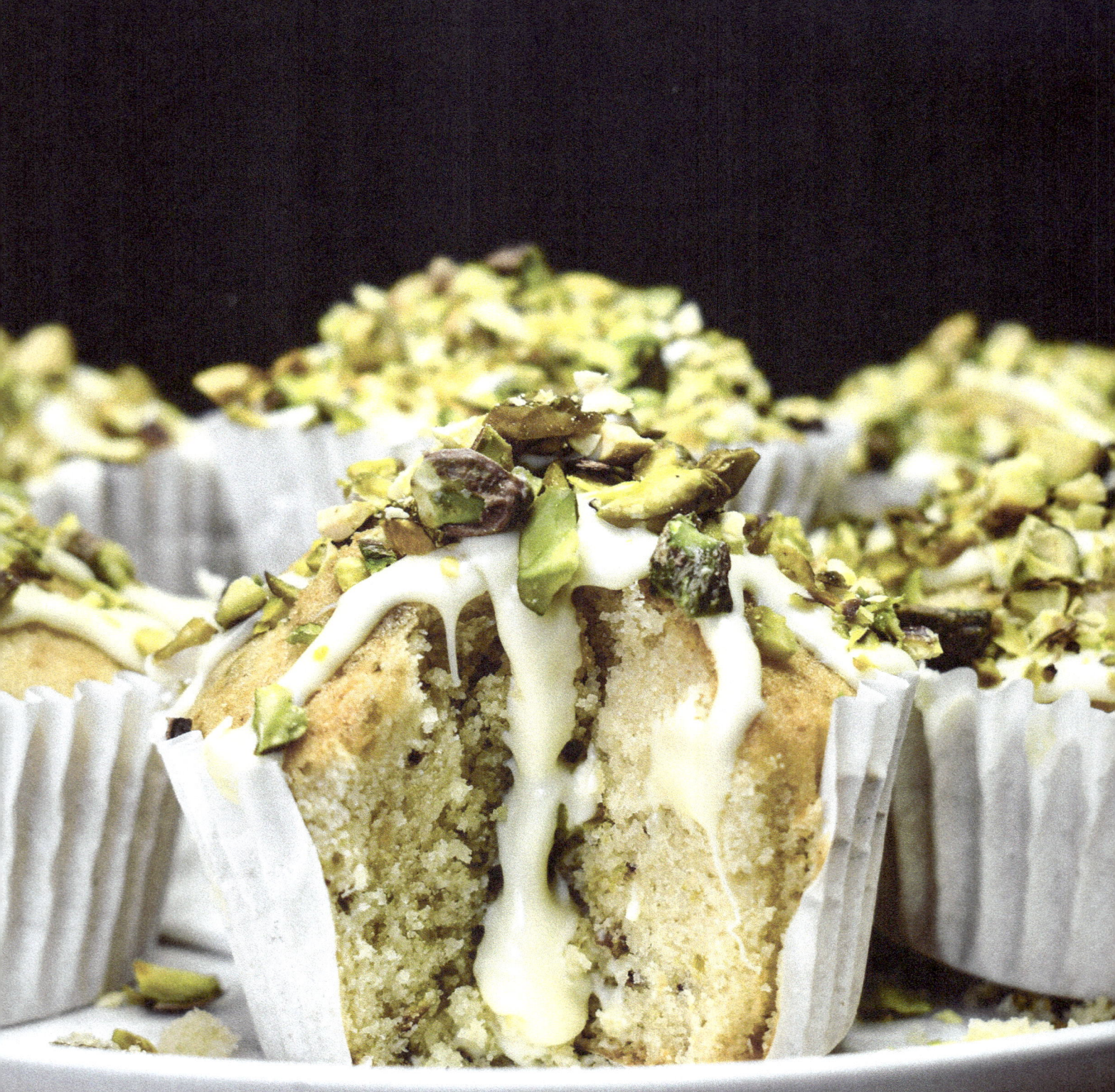

PISTACHIO WHITE CHOCOLATE CUPCAKES

Ingredients

225g (1½ cups) plain flour
110g (½ cup) granulated sugar
110g (½ cup) light brown sugar
½ tsp baking powder
¼ tsp baking soda
¼ tsp salt
2 large eggs - *at room temperature*
113g (½ cup) unsalted butter - *melted*
125g (½ cup) plain yogurt
63 ml (¼ cup) milk - *at room temperature*
1 tsp vanilla extract
100g shelled pistachio - *finally chopped*
190g (1 cup) white chocolate chips - *melted for garnish*

Method

1. Preheat oven to 170°C fan-forced and line a 12 cupcakes pan with paper liners.

2. In a large bowl, whisk together the flour, granulated sugar, brown sugar, baking powder, baking soda, and salt.

3. In another bowl, combined melted butter, eggs, yogurt, milk and vanilla extract.

4. Add the wet ingredients to the dry ingredients and mix until just combined, then fold in the chopped pistachios.

5. Divide the mix evenly among the paper liners. Bake for 18-20 minutes

6. Let the cupcakes cool for 5 minutes, then transfer to a wire rack to cool completely

7. Drizzle the melted white chocolate and sprinkle with additional chopped pistachios as desired.

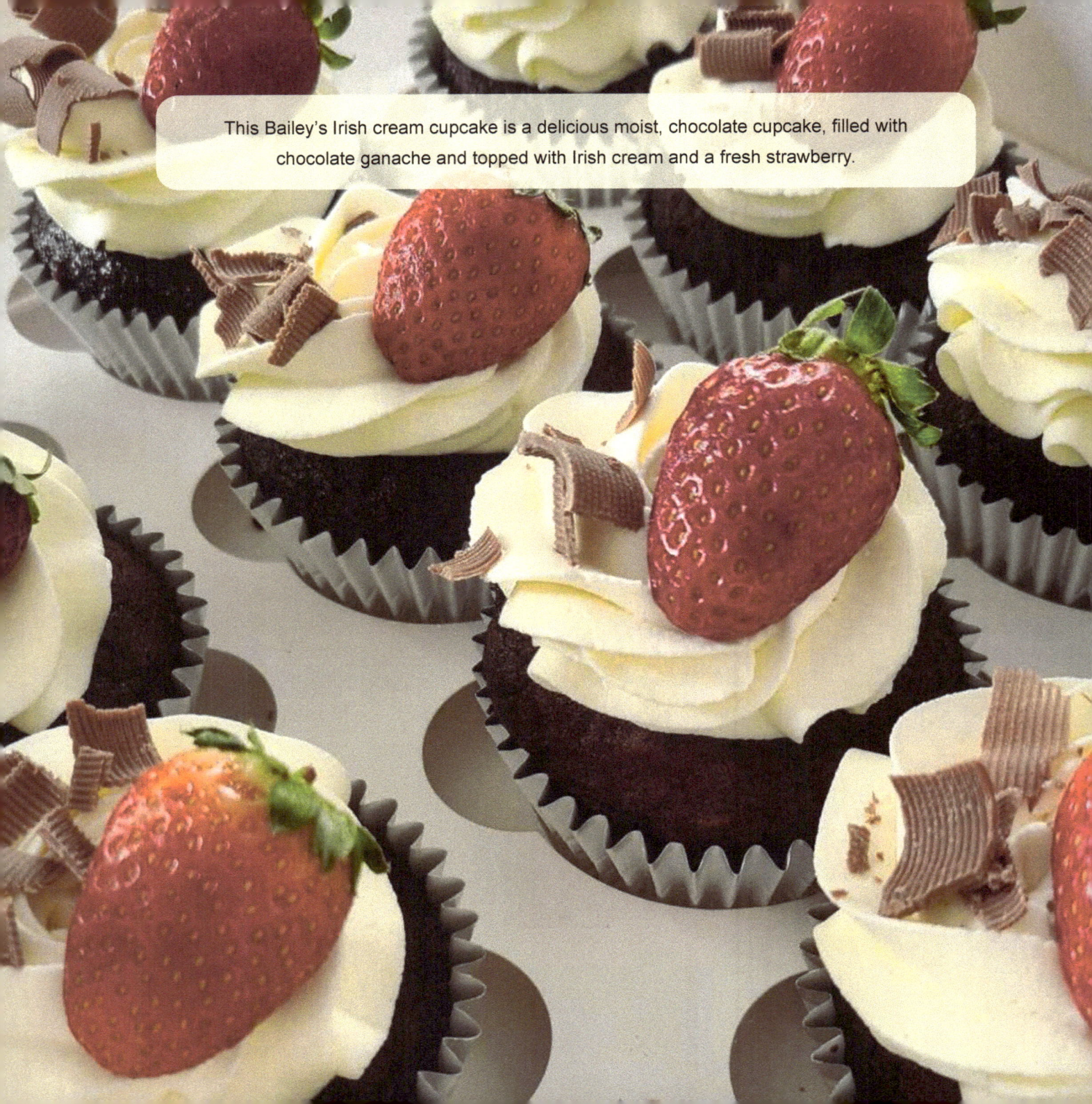

This Bailey's Irish cream cupcake is a delicious moist, chocolate cupcake, filled with chocolate ganache and topped with Irish cream and a fresh strawberry.

CREAMY, DREAMY IRISH DELIGHTS

Ingredients

Cupcakes

188g (1¼ cups) flour

50g (½ cup) cocoa powder - *unsweetened*

2 tsp espresso powder

1½ tsp baking powder

½ tsp salt

120ml (½ cup) vegetable oil

220g (1 cup) caster sugar

2 large eggs - *room temperature*

¼ cup brewed espresso or coffee

2 tbsp Bailey's Irish Cream

Topping

225g (1 cup) unsalted butter - *at room temperature*

320g (2 cups) soft icing sugar

¼ tsp salt

3 tbsp Bailey's Irish Cream

Chocolate ganache

120g dark chocolate, *finely chopped*

125ml (½ cup) thickened cream

1 tbsp Bailey's Irish Cream

Method

Chocolate ganache

1. Finely chop the dark chocolate and place into a large glass bowl.
2. Place the heavy cream in microwave safe bowl and microwave for 1-2 minute.
3. Pour over the chopped chocolate and let it sit for about 3 minutes.
4. Using a spatula, gently mix until chocolate is fully melted and fully combined and smooth. Add Irish Cream and mix until combined.
5. Let it sit in the fridge until it thickens enough to hold its shape.

Cupcakes

6. Preheat oven to 170 °C fan forced.
7. In a small bowl, whisk flour, cocoa powder, espresso coffee, baking powder and salt. Set aside.
8. In a large bowl, whisk vegetable oil and caster sugar until fully combined. Then whisk in the eggs until smooth. Add the brewed espresso and Irish cream and whisk until combined.
9. Then gently mix in the dry ingredients until fully incorporated - the batter will be thin.
10. Pour into the cupcake's liner about halfway full.
11. Bake for about 20-22 minutes or until skewer comes out clean.
12. Remove from pan and let cool in wire rack.
13. Let the chocolate cupcakes cool completely, before filling and frosting
14. Use a cupcake corer, to remove the centre of each cupcake, then fill with 2 tbsp of chocolate ganache.

Frosting

15. In a large bowl using a mixer, fitted with a paddle attachment, cream butter and icing sugar until smooth.
16. Set the mixer to low speed and slowly drizzle the Irish cream until fully incorporated, then add the salt and beat the frosting on high for 5 minutes until light and fluffy.
17. Frost the filled Irish cream chocolate cupcakes and garnish with fresh a strawberry, chocolate swirl, or according to your desired preference.

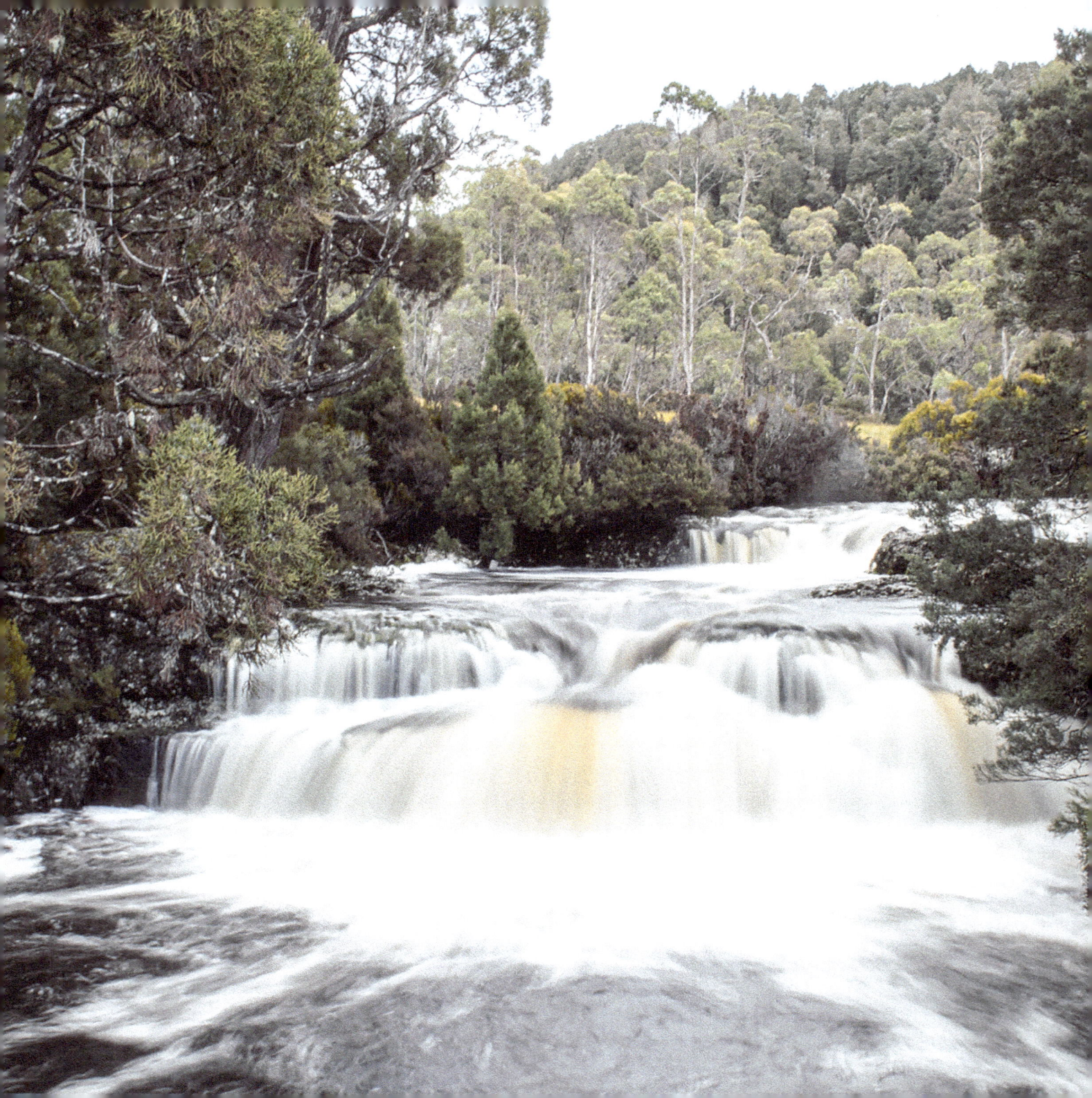

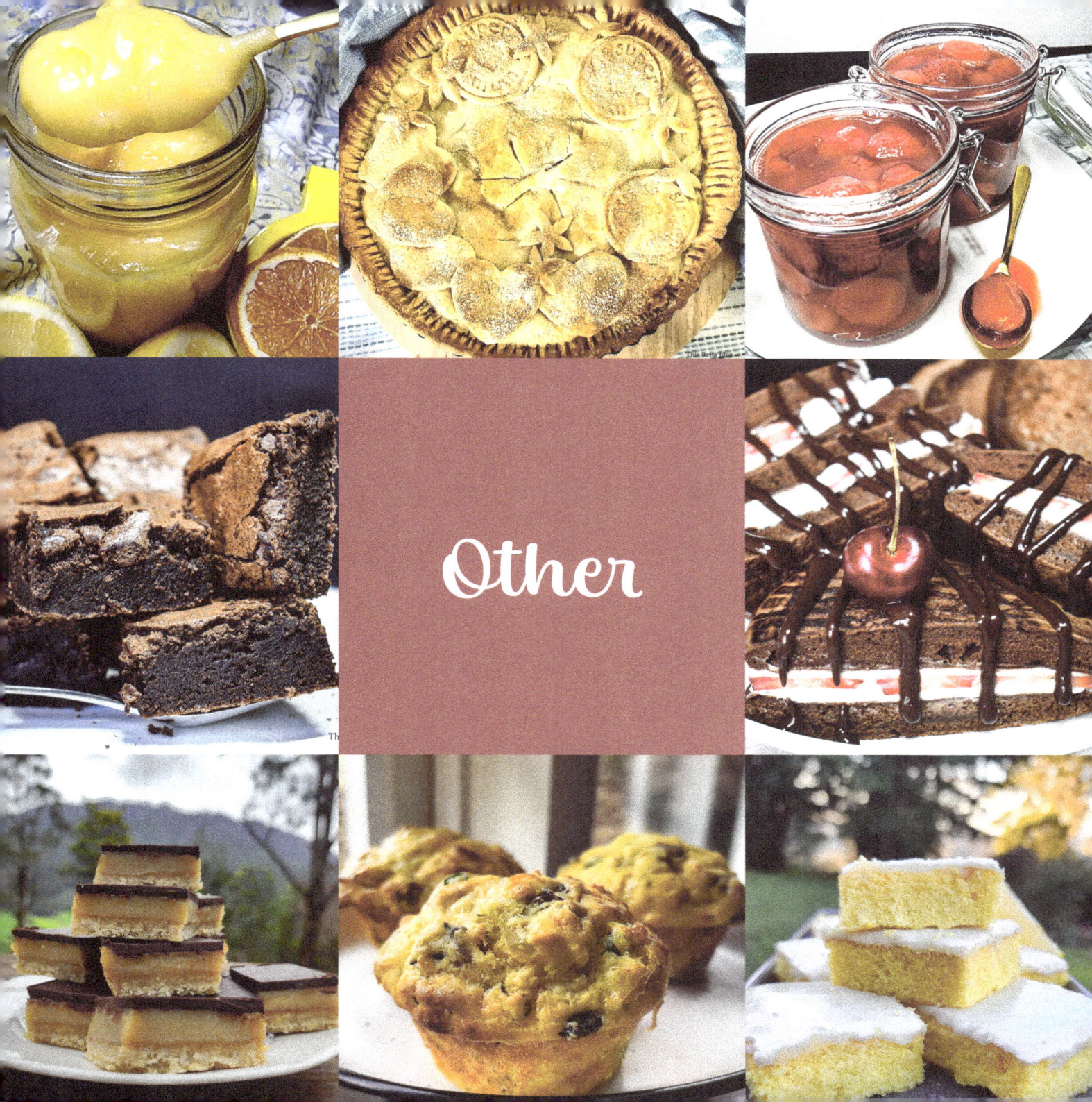

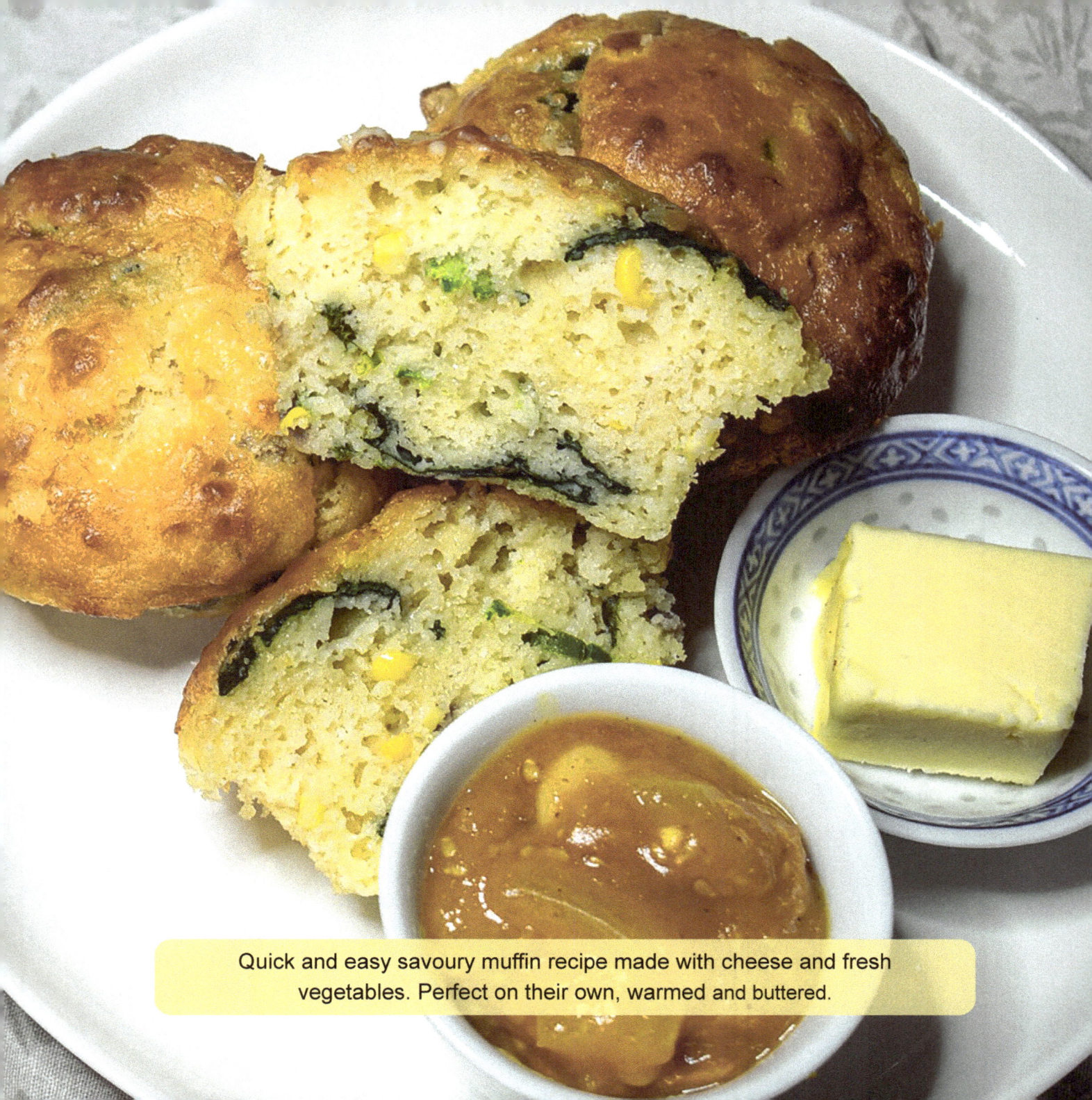
Quick and easy savoury muffin recipe made with cheese and fresh vegetables. Perfect on their own, warmed and buttered.

SAVOURY MUFFINS

Ingredients

Dry ingredients

225g (1½ cups) self-raising flour
1 tsp baking powder
1 tsp salt
250g (2 cups) grated cheddar cheese

Wet Ingredients

63ml (¼ cup) plain yogurt - *room temperature*
2 eggs beaten - *room temperature*
250ml (1 cup) milk - *room temperature*
100ml (0.4 cup) vegetable oil
2 tbsp oil - *for brushing pan*

Optional

Spring onion, red onion, mushroom, spinach. Sauté for about 3 minutes and set to cool

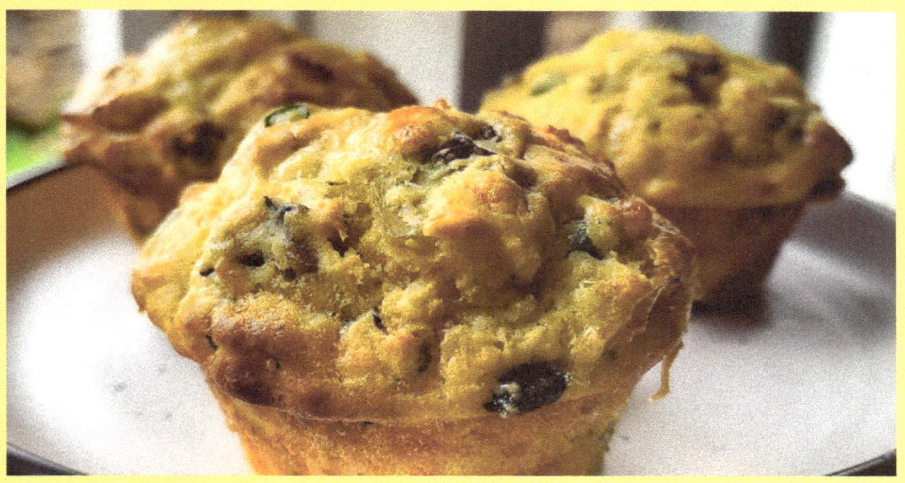

Method

1. Preheat oven to 180 °C fan forced. Brush the inside of muffin pan with oil
2. Mix the dry ingredients in a medium bowl, sifting well
3. Mix the wet ingredients in another bowl, stirring until well combined
4. Add the wet mixture to the dry ingredients. Also add the sauté vegetables here as well (should be completely cooled). Mix until completely well combined, but don't over mix
5. Scoop into each of the 12 muffins forms and bake for 20-25 minutes
6. Serve warm with butter and/or tomato relish

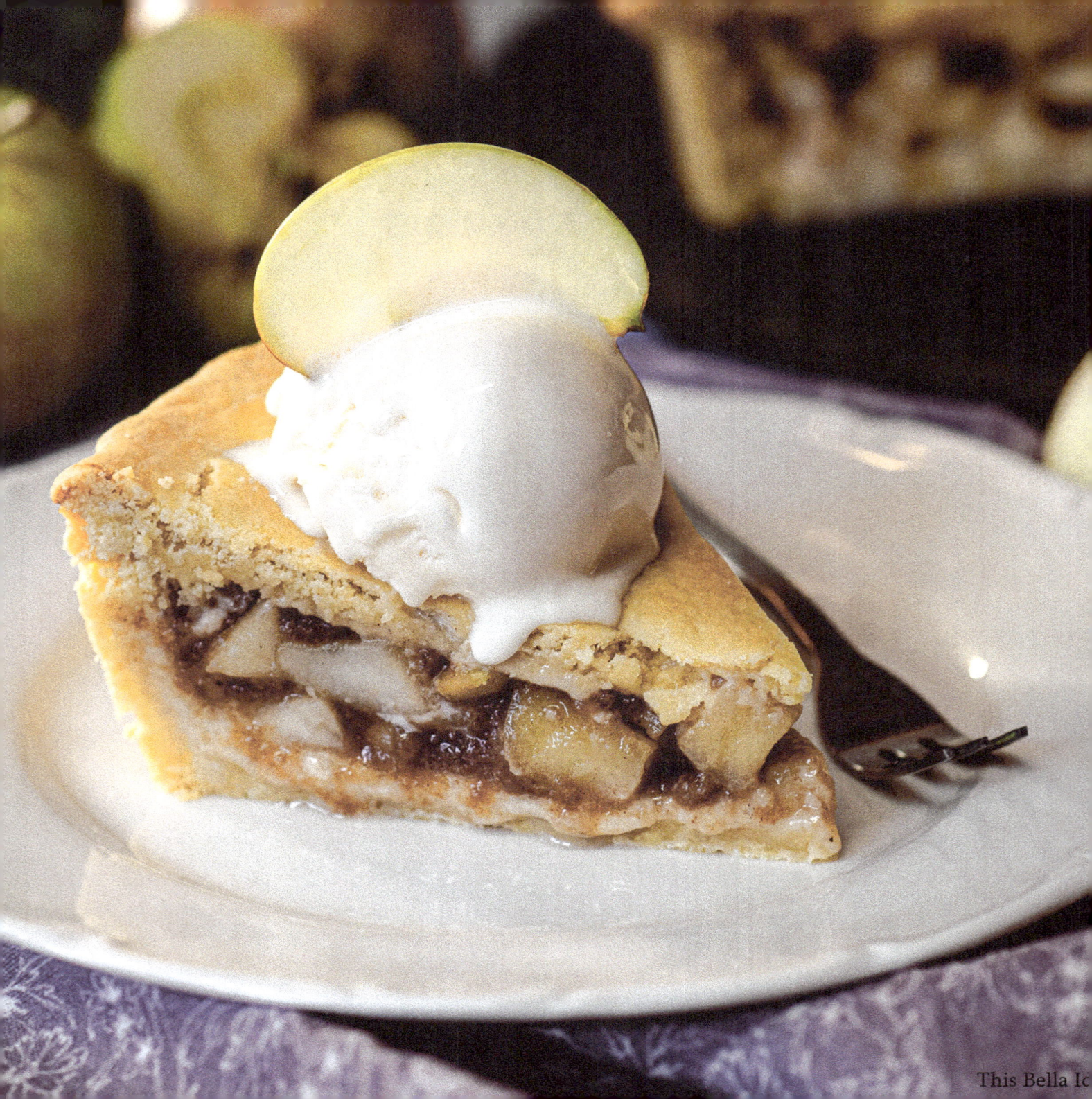

APPLE PIE

Ingredients

The filling

600g (8 large) granny Smith apples - *peeled, cored and cut into 1 cm cubes.*
55g (¼ cup) white granulated sugar – *more or less according to taste*
3 tsp lemon juice
1 tsp cinnamon ground
¼ tsp ground cloves
3 tsp cornflour (cornstarch) - *mixed to a paste with 40 ml cold water.*

The Pastry

113g (½ cup) salted butter - *very soft*
145g (⅔ cup) white granulated sugar
150g (1 cup) self-raising flour
300g (2 cups) pastry flour - *or you can use plain flour.*
2 eggs - *at room temperature*
1 tsp baking soda
Ice cream to serve

Method

Making the filling

1. Place the apples in a saucepan with 60 ml water, bring to boil and then reduce the heat and simmer until the apples is just tender.
2. Stir in the sugar, ground cinnamon, ground cloves and lemon juice. While still simmering, gradually stir in the cornflour paste. It should create a thick custard consistency.

Making the pastry

3. Using the hand whisk, mix the butter and sugar until creamy, then whisk in the eggs until well combined.
4. In a separate bowl, sift the dry ingredients. Then using a large metal spoon, fold this into the egg mixture until well combined. Cover and set aside while waiting for the filling to cool.

Assembly

5. Roll out the large pastry ball on a floured workbench to about a 30cm circle (about 2 mm thick). Roll the pastry around rolling pin and then unroll over a 22cm round metal pie dish. Gently press into corners and allow extra for some overhang. Place the filling in the base. Roll the small pastry piece to 25 cm circle.
6. Lift the pie dish and cut the excess from around edges with sharp knife. Chill for 30 minutes.
7. Preheat oven to 180 °C fan forced. Place pie dish into baking tray and cut air vents in the centre of the pie. Bake for 45 minutes or until golden brown.
8. Serve either warm or cold with ice cream.

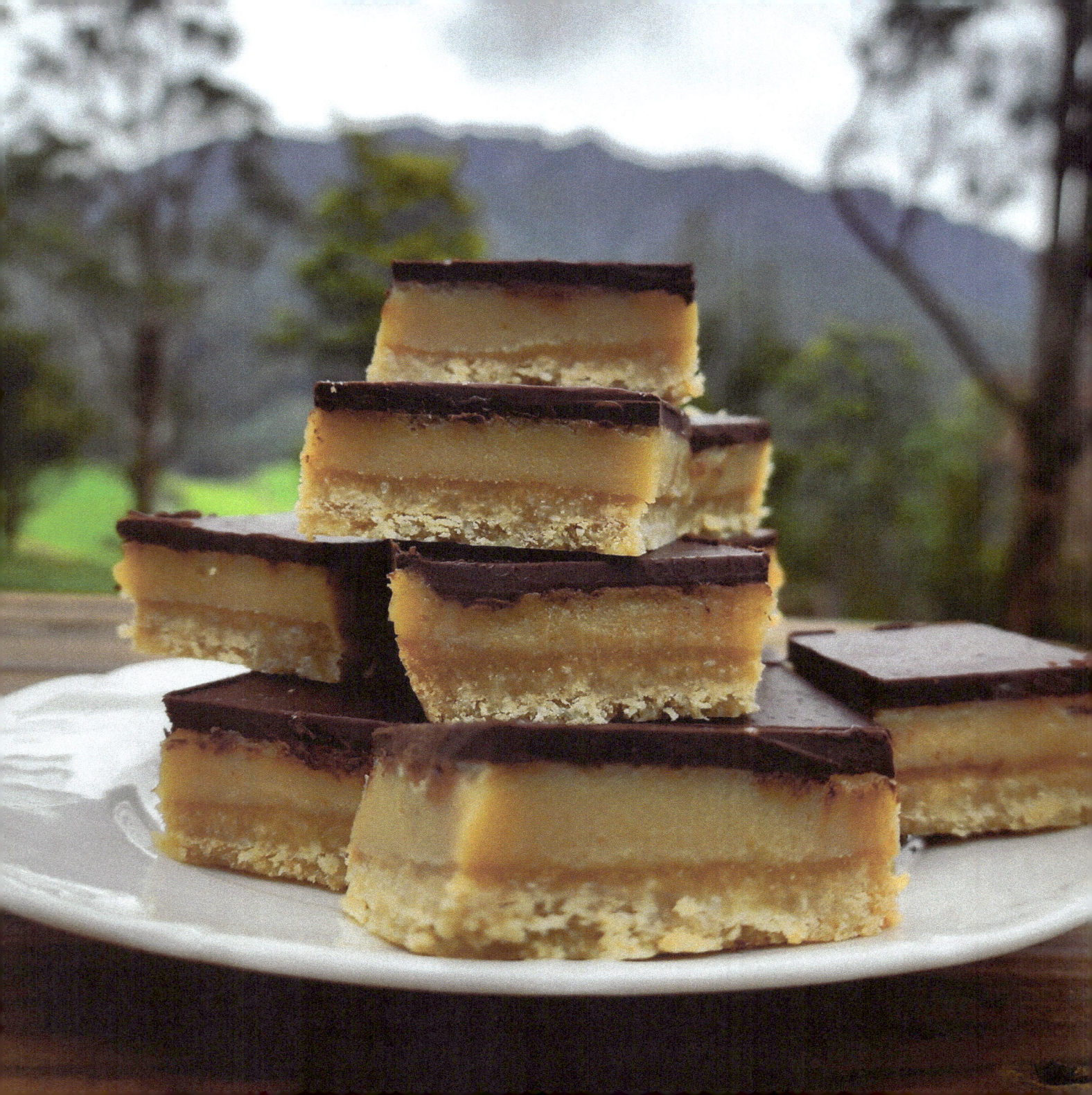

CARAMEL SLICE

Ingredients

Base

150g (1 cup) all-purpose flour
110g (½ cup) brown sugar
43g (½ cup) desiccated coconut
113g (½ cup) unsalted butter - *melted*

Caramel Filling

113g (½ cup) unsalted butter
110g (½ cup) brown sugar
1 tsp vanilla extract
1 tin (395g) sweetened condensed milk

Chocolate Topping

200g dark chocolate - *broken into small pieces*
1 tbsp vegetable oil

Method

1. Preheat fan forced oven to 160 C
2. Grease and line a 28 x 18 cm baking dish with overhanging parchment paper
3. Mix all base ingredients until well combined
4. Press mixture into prepared dish
5. Bake for 15 minutes or until golden
6. Prepare caramel filling (steps below)
7. Pour caramel over baked base
8. Refrigerate until set
9. Melt chocolate topping (steps below)
10. Spread over caramel layer
11. Refrigerate until chocolate sets

Caramel filling: Melt butter and brown sugar in a saucepan over medium heat. Add vanilla extract. Pour condensed milk. Stir constantly until caramel thickens.

Chocolate topping: Melt chocolate in a double boiler or microwave (30 second intervals). Stir in vegetable oil

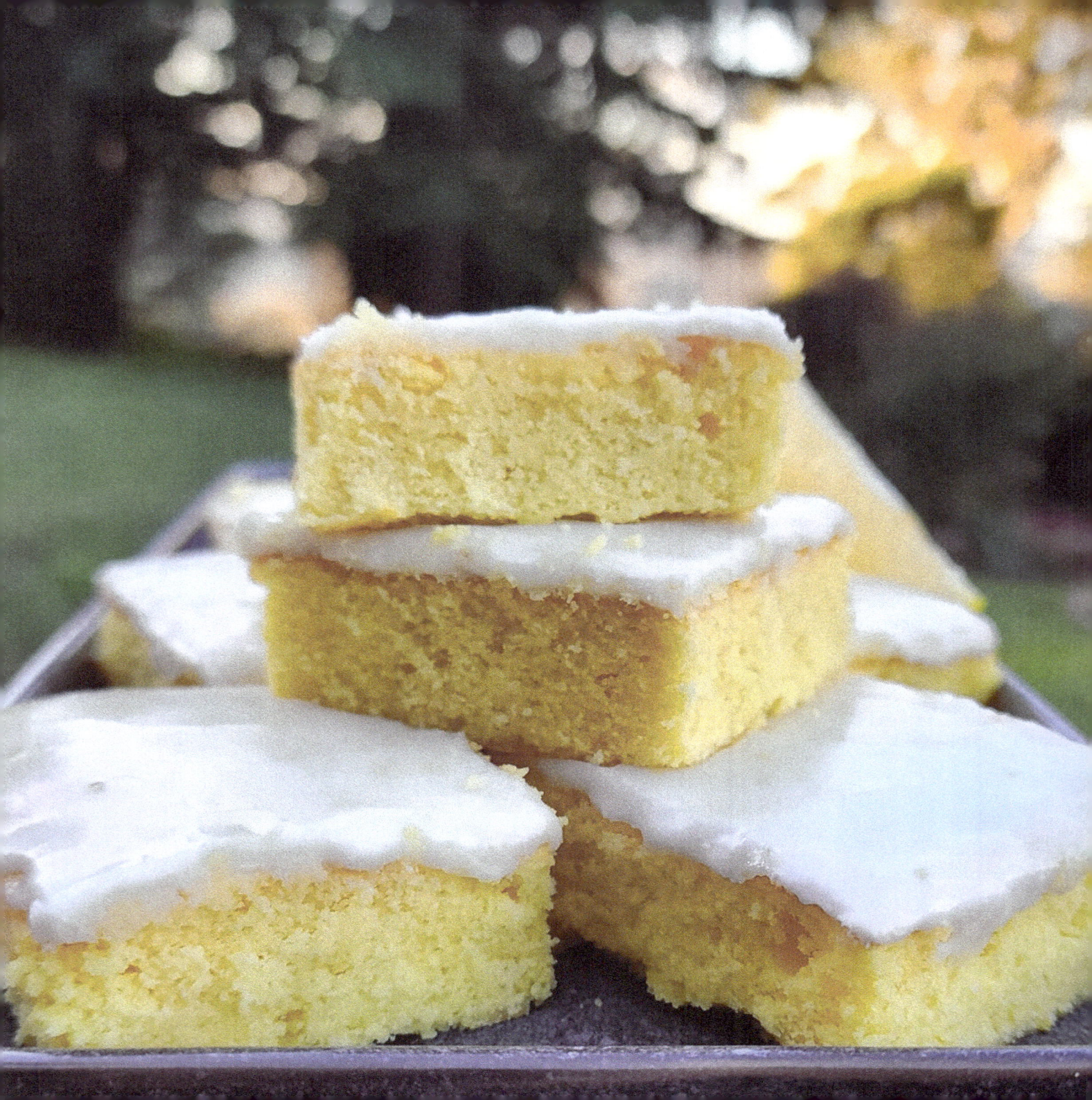

SUNSHINE IN A SQUARE

Taste the sunshine in every bite of our lemon brownies-zesty, tangy, and irresistibly addictive!

Ingredients

220g (1 cup) granulated sugar
113g (½ cup) unsalted butter - *in room temperature*
2 large eggs
1 large lemon - *just for the zest*
4 tbsp lemon juice
188g (1¼ cups) flour
½ tsp salt

Glaze

160g (1 cup) powdered sugar
2-3 tbsp lemon juice
Zest of one lemon

Method

1. Preheat oven to 160°C fan forced. Line an 8" x 8" baking pan with parchment or foil and spray with nonstick spray

2. Cream the butter and sugar until light and fluffy. Blend the eggs, one at the time, while mixing in the lemon zest and juice. Stir in the salt and fold in the flour, stirring just until everything is well incorporated.

3. Pour the batter into the pan and smooth it out evenly

4. Bake for 20 minutes, or until a skewer comes out clean. Allow to cool

Making the zest

5. In a small bowl, whisk together powdered sugar and lemon juice and zest until spreadable. Pour over the bars and smooth out. Let the glaze set, then cut into squares and serve.

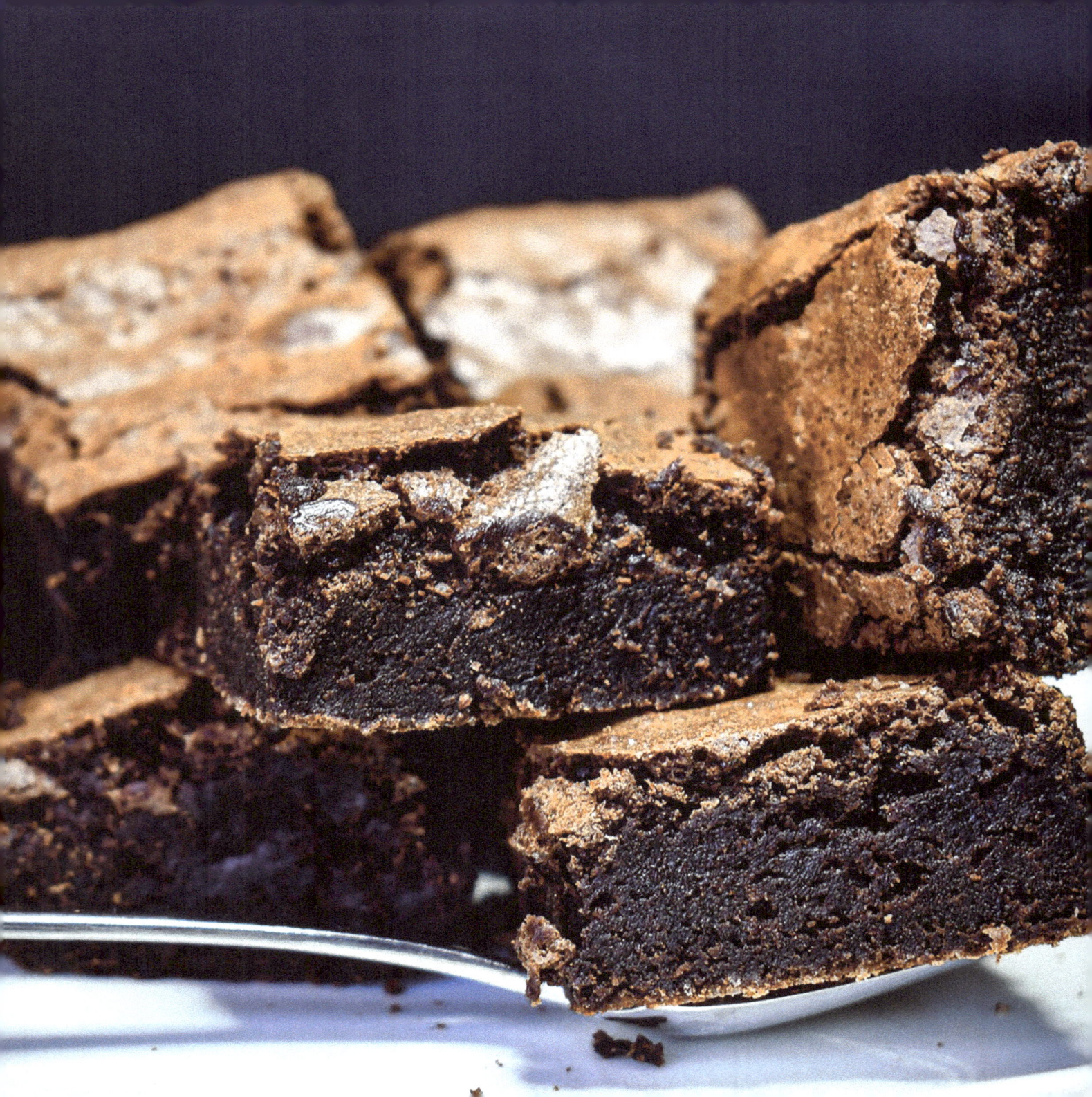

BROWNIES

This is a simple brownie recipe, made with common kitchen ingredients. Soft and gooey inside while crisp and crackly on top

Ingredients

365g (1⅔ cups) of granulated sugar
188g (1¼ cups) plain flour
225g (1 cup) unsalted butter
3 eggs - *at room temperature*
50g (½ cup) Cocoa powder
1 tsp vanilla extract
½ tsp baking powder
¼ tsp salt

Method

1. Preheat oven to 170°C fan forced. Grease a 9 x 13-inch pan

2. Mix sugar, flour, melted butter, eggs, cocoa powder, vanilla, baking powder and salt in a large bowl until combined. Spread evenly into the prepared pan.

3. Bake in the preheated oven until top is dry and edges have started to pull away from the sides of the pan. Approximately 35 to 40 minutes.

4. Cool before slicing into squares.

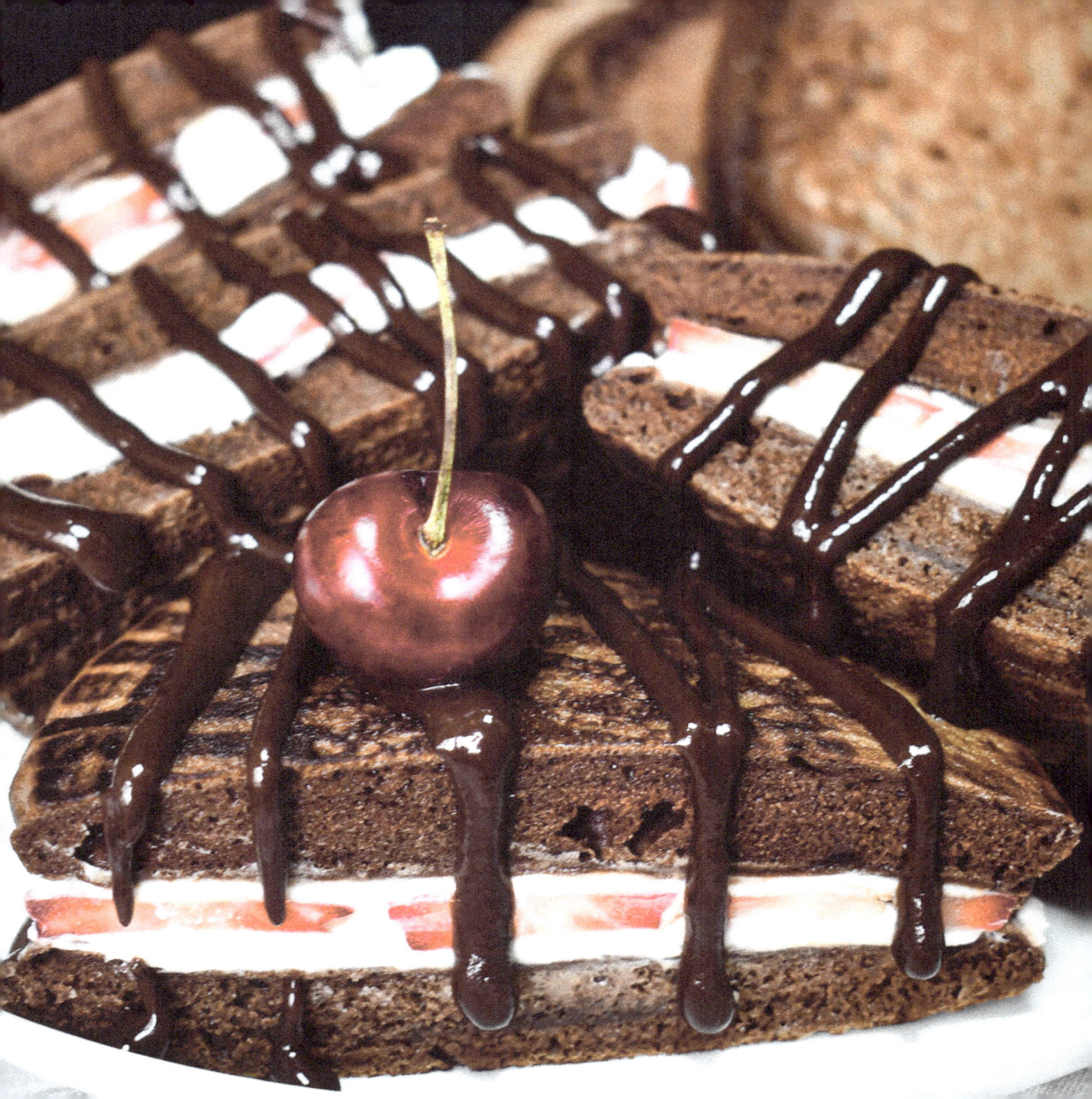

EGGLESS CHOCOLATE PANCAKES

Simple, easy to make, soft and fluffy, not too sweet and healthy

Ingredients

150g (1 cup) flour
38g (¼ cup) chocolate powder
½ tsp baking soda
80g (½ cup) icing sugar
25g (¼ cup) milk powder
1 tbsp vegetable oil
¼ tsp salt
250ml (1 cup) butter milk (1 cup milk + 1 tsp vinegar) - *in room temperature*

Method

1. Mix well together flour, chocolate powder, baking soda, icing sugar, milk powder, salt.

2. Add butter milk to the flour mixture and stir until well combined

3. Prepared a nonstick frypan on medium heat.

4. Pour a scoop the batter into the pan, cook until bubbles form and edges are dry. Flip and cook until brown on the other side. Repeat for the remaining batter

5. To assemble, create a sandwich with 2 chocolate pancakes spread with chocolate ganache and garnish with a fresh strawberry.

THE BEST LEMON CURD

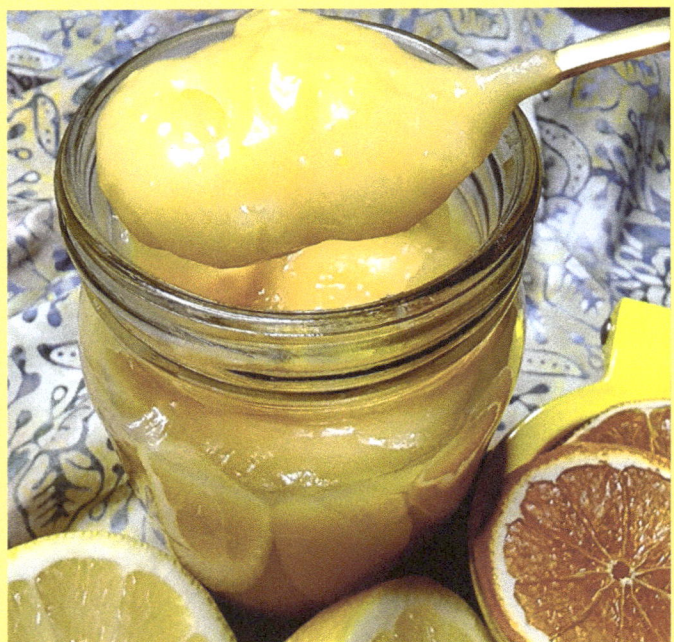

This is a simple and easy recipe, resulting in the perfect lemon curd for spreading on cookies, cakes, breads and pies.

Ingredients

5 large eggs - *at room temperature*
240g (1 cup) freshly squeezed lemon juice
220g (1 cup) granulated sugar
6-8 lemon zest
113g (½ cup) of unsalted butter - *at room temperature*
¼ tsp salt

Method

1. Place the sugar in a medium sized pot and mix in lemon zest and whisk together.

2. Pour the lemon juice into the pot and gently stir in the sugar.

3. In another bowl, crack all the eggs and add salt. Beat thoroughly using a hand mixer or fork

4. Pour the eggs into the sugar mix and whisk well. Set the pot over the low heat.

5. Allow to cook, stirring constantly until the curd thickens, or until it coats to the rubber spatula. You'll know the consistency is correct if the curd on the spatula does not fold back together when separated with your finger.

6. Pour the curd through a sieve (to remove the zest) into a bowl containing the butter. Stir until the butter is thoroughly melted.

7. Pour the curd into an airtight container and store in the fridge.

TWO INGREDIENTS CHOCOLATE GANACHE

Ingredients

350g (2 cups) dark chocolate chips
188ml (¾ cup) thickened cream

Method

1. In a microwave safe bowl, add dark chocolate chips and thickened cream
2. Microwave on high for 1 minute and 10 seconds
3. Whisk together until completely combined
4. Store in refrigerator until ready to use.

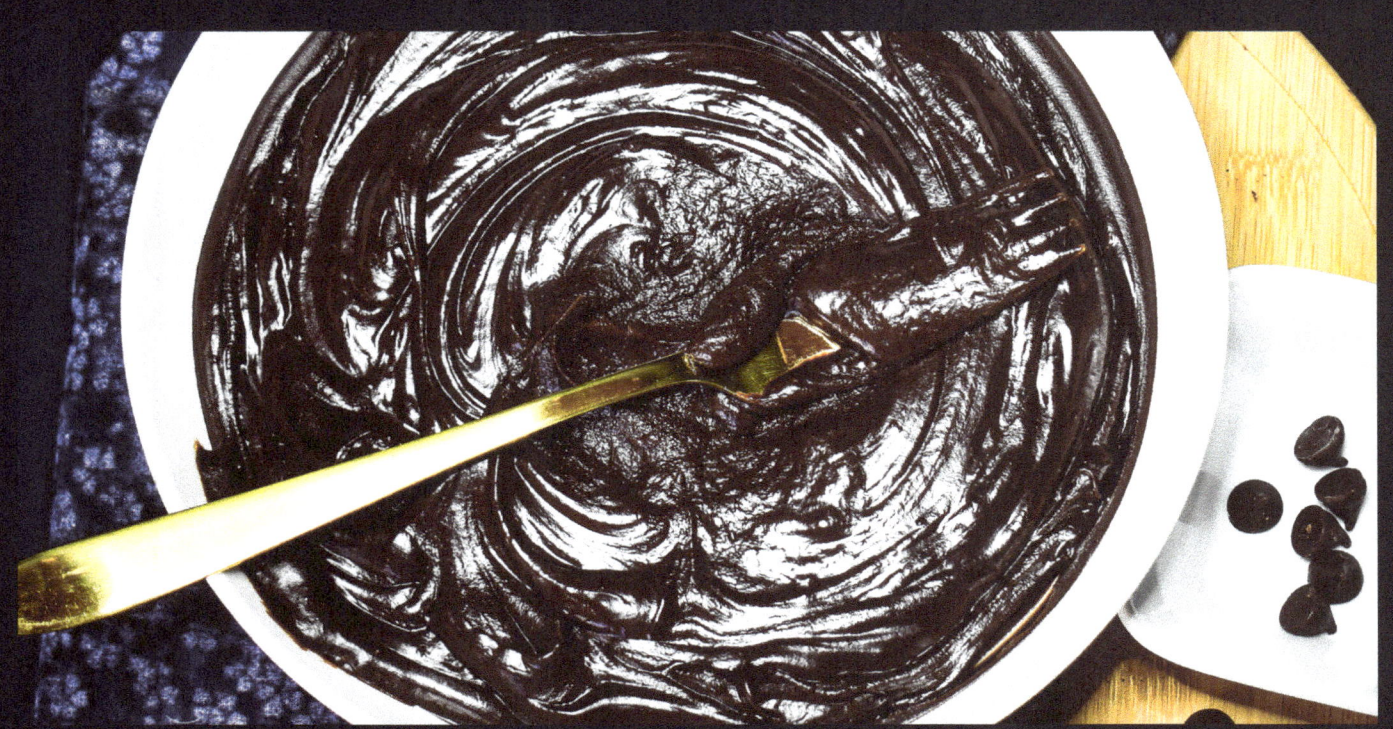

WHITE CHOCOLATE GANACHE

This light and fluffy buttercream is super stable, makes a great cake filling and frosting, and is excellent for piping decorations.

Ingredients

Frosting

190g (1 cup) finely chopped white chocolate, or white chocolate chips
83g (⅓ cup) thickened cream - *I use Bulla*

Method

1. Place white chocolate in a medium size bowl and set aside
2. Pour the thickened cream into a heat proof bowl and heat, in 15 second intervals, in the microwave until it just begins to bubble (it will usually take about a minute)
3. Pour the thickened cream over the white chocolate and let the mixture sit for a couple of minutes
4. Using a spatula, mix the ganache until the mixture has come together and is smooth. Press a piece of plastic wrap flush against the ganache, and place the bowl in the fridge to chill.
5. When the ganache is ready to use, you can put it in piping bag fitted with a large round piping tip. The consistency should be thick enough to scoop into the piping bag and hold its shape.

CHOCOLATE SHARDS

Simple ingredients list, yet impressive outcome

Ingredients

High-quality dark chocolate

Method

1. Melt chocolate to perfection
2. Temper for rich, glossy finish
3. Pour onto parchment paper or silicone mat (I use a spoon to create single shards)
4. Allow to set, then break into delicate shards

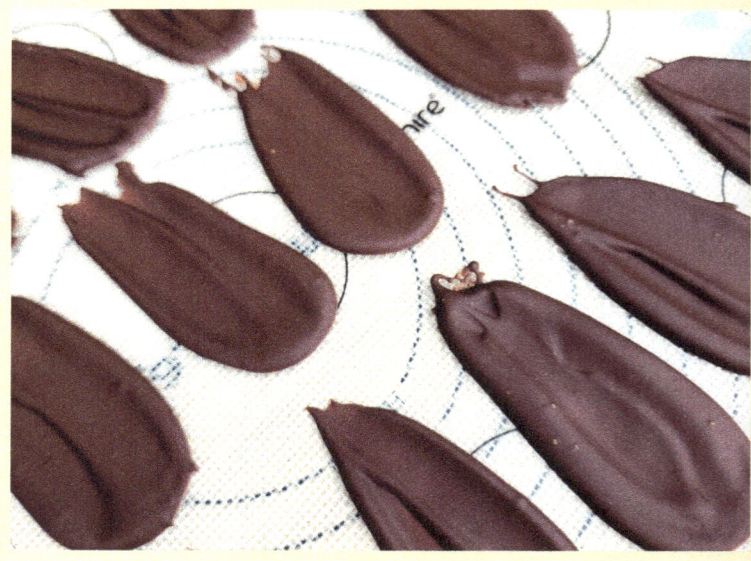

STRAWBERRY COMPOTE

Strawberry compote is so easy to make, all you need is fresh frozen strawberries, a bit of sugar, and a splash of water or juice. Use strawberry compote just like you'd use jam or other fillings for cakes or cupcakes.

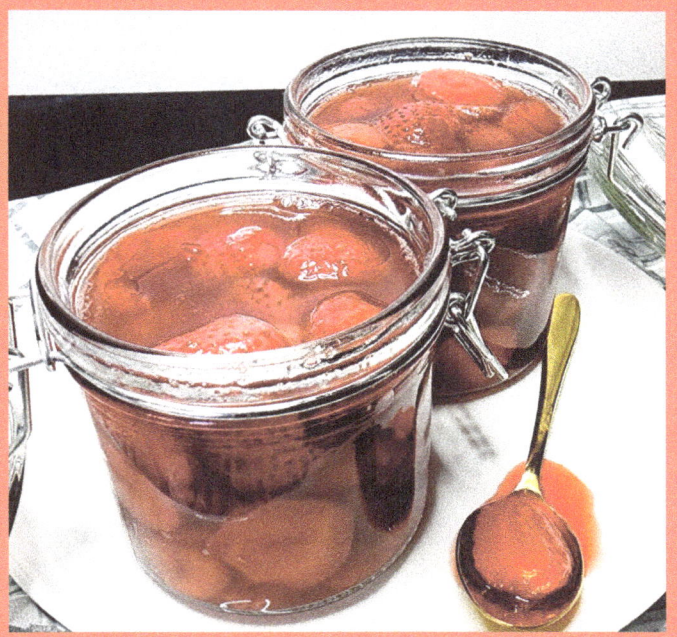

Ingredients

500g fresh or frozen strawberries
55g (¼ cup) of sugar
1 tbsp fresh lemon juice
½ tbsp vanilla extract
1 tsp corn starch + 2 tsp water for making slurry

Method

1. Combine strawberries, sugar, vanilla and lemon juice in saucepan.

2. Bring to simmer over a medium heat and stirring occasionally or until the strawberries are soft and juicy and then add the slurry

3. Remove from the heat. Compote will be thickened when it's cold.

BUTTER CREAM

Ingredients

Frosting

150g (⅔ cup) slightly salted butter - *softened*

240g (1½ cups) icing sugar

1 tbsp milk

Method

1. Using an electric mixer, beat the butter in a bowl until pale, gradually add icing sugar and milk, beating constantly until combined.

ITALIAN BUTTER CREAM

This light and fluffy buttercream is super stable, makes a great cake filling and frosting, and is excellent for piping decorations.

Ingredients

Frosting

4 large egg whites

275g (1¼ cups) sugar

¼ tsp salt

450g (2 cups) unsalted butter - *at room temperature*

1 tsp vanilla extract

Method

1. Place the egg whites and ¼ of the sugar in electric mixer fitted with the whisk attachment.

2. Beat on medium to speed until the egg whites reach the soft peak stage.

3. Meanwhile pour the remaining sugar and 75ml of water in medium sized saucepan set over the medium heat. Attach a candy thermometer to the side of pan and bring to the soft-ball stage, without stirring at 120 °C

4. Continue to whip the egg whites on medium to high speed and slowly drizzle in the hot syrup until the bottom of the bowl and the mixture is cool. This takes about 10 minutes. The mixture should be thick with firm peaks at this point. Beat in the salt.

5. While still beating at medium to high speed, add the butter - a few pieces at a time. The butter cream may appear to thin out somewhat, but it will thicken into firm peaks once all the butter is added. Beat in the vanilla extract. If the butter is still loose, continue to beat on high speed until it is thickened.

FRESH CREAM FROSTING

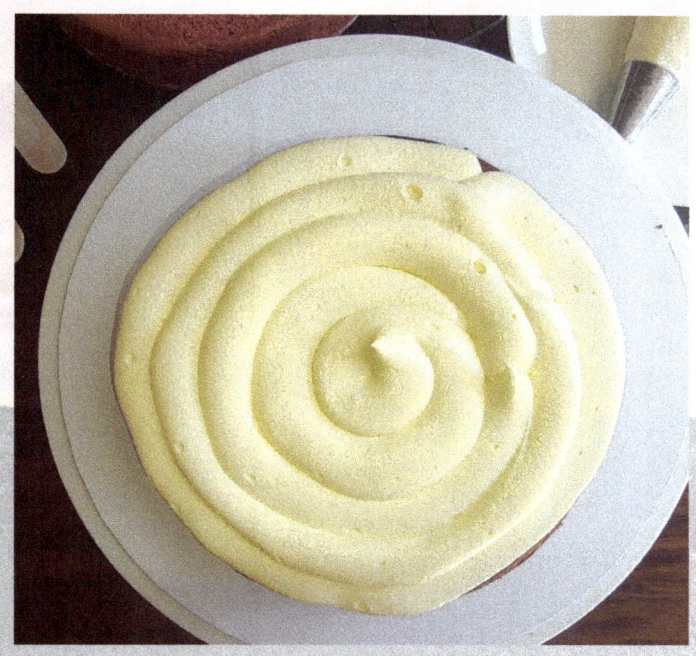

Ingredients

750ml (3 cups) thickened cream
2 tsp vanilla
7 tbsp powdered sugar
2 tbsp milk powder

Method

1. In the large mixing bowl add thickened cream, sugar, milk powder, vanilla and whisk with electric mixer for 3 -5 minutes until stiff peaks
2. Pipe the frosting onto the cake

CREAM CHEESE DIP

Ingredients

250g Philadelphia cream cheese
250ml (1 cup) sour cream
1 tbsp Dijon mustard
½ tsp garlic powder
½ tsp onion powder
½ tsp smoked paprika
250g (2 cups) shredded cheddar cheese
2 tbsp white wine

Method

1. Place the cream cheese on a microwave safe plate, soften in the microwave for 10 seconds.
2. Using a rubber spatula, mix until soften and fluffy.
3. Place the softened cream cheese into a bowl. Add sour cream, Dijon mustard, garlic powder, onion powder, smoked paprika, white wine. The add the shredded cheese and mix to combine
4. Allow the dip rest for 30 minutes before serving.

LEMON BUTTER CREAM

Zesty flavour, rich, creamy butter – a stable lemon delight – delicious!

Ingredients

3 egg whites - *at room temperature*

220g (1 cup) caster sugar

225g unsalted butter - *soft*

2 tsp lemon juice

¼ tsp lemon zest

Method

1. Mix together egg whites and sugar with a spoon or fork until well combined.
2. Put in microwave for 10 second intervals until you don't feel the sugar when you touch the mixture. (be careful that you don't let the white eggs cook)
3. While still warm, transfer to a mixing bowl with the whisk attached. Mix until super firm, stiff peak, meringue
4. Change the whisk with paddle attachment and add the soft butter, little by little
5. When the butter starts to get creamy, add lemon juice and lemon zest.
6. Your lemon butter cream ready to use for your lemon cake or lemon cupcakes.

www.ingramcontent.com/pod-product-compliance
Lightning Source LLC
Chambersburg PA
CBHW042358070526
44585CB00029B/2983